Fireside Wisdom

*Conversations to Inspire
Personal Mastery*

Also by Roddy Carter

BodyWHealth: Journey to Abundance

BodyWHealth: Invitation

Sunset Lessons: Reflections on Light and Love from the Darkest of Places

Fireside Wisdom

Conversations to Inspire Personal Mastery

Roddy Carter, MD

Aquila Life Science Press
La Jolla, California

FIRST AQUILA LIFE SCIENCE PRESS EDITION, NOVEMBER 2021
Published by Aquila Life Science, LLC, La Jolla, CA

FIRESIDE WISDOM.

ISBN: 978-0-9969889-7-1

Printed in the United States of America

With deep appreciation

for all the fellow travelers

who have kindly shared

their curiosity and wisdom,

sometimes in silence,

as we have sat together

inspired and uplifted

beside the great fire of life.

CONTENTS

ACKNOWLEDGEMENTS

To my family and friends, my mentors and colleagues, my patients and clients, and the countless authors I have not met whose contagious wisdom has generously filled the pages of a thousand books, I am truly grateful.

Sarah Dawson has been an invaluable companion through this journey. As she did with my earlier books, she has worked with unflagging enthusiasm and quiet diplomacy to bring her editing genius to this third work. She wields two gifts that are rarely found together: a commanding overview, and an extraordinary eye for detail. Sarah, I am truly grateful for the love and support you have brought to this book, and to the mission it represents—the sharing of wisdom!

Jolie Kalfaian brings her superior artistic talents to the design and layout of *Fireside Wisdom*, as she did with my first two books. She integrates practical design that makes the work easier to read with uplifting creativity that makes it a work of beauty. This is the nature of wisdom, both useful and inspiring. Thank you, Jolie; I am truly proud of both the look and the feel of *Fireside Wisdom*.

PREFACE

I have been gifted with great wisdom—not my own, I hasten to add.

No, I have been gifted with a seemingly endless stream of occasions where life has revealed deep insights to me. This happens during chance conversations, reflective walks on the beach, idle daydreaming, and unexpected moments while we are busy with the serious work of living. And my favorites…those have arrived with good friends alongside a hearty fire!

For some reason, not everyone seems to receive these powerful insights. I believe that we have to be looking for them to see them. When we are open to them, we recognize that they are, in fact, the wisdom we strive so hard to acquire throughout our lifetimes. I am lucky and truly grateful to see them.

I have always been curious. As long as I can remember, I have been earnestly seeking truth, desiring to understand who we are, how we work, and within what larger context we operate. How else could a creative humanitarian have pursued the rigors of science with such vigorous determination?

But it's the outer frontiers of knowledge, where the shadows cast by the great fire dance alluringly, that have inspired me most. Unlike many scientists who live in fear of the unknown, I have been drawn to it. It is this magnetic pull that has fueled my own passionate journey of self-discovery, self-optimization, and, ultimately, self-mastery.

Many of the insights that I share in this collection come from my fascination with our natural evolution that has resulted in our magnificent neuro-psychobiology.

As a young man studying medicine in Africa, I would travel with friends into remote wilderness areas to explore nature in its most pristine and untouched state. This afforded me uniquely powerful vistas of primal life—a life relatively free of the fingerprints of modern *Homo sapiens*. You can't watch a lioness taking down a buffalo to feed her children or a giraffe giving birth without developing a deep appreciation for our natural design, and for the extraordinary pathway that has led us toward who we are and the life we live today.

At the fireside at the end of each day, with the sound of cackling jackals, roaring lions, and the magical song of African nightjars in the background, we gathered in deep discourse. We sat together, young men and women with their full adult lives ahead, in earnest reverence for the universe that presented us with this wonderful invitation, called life. Perhaps it was there, alongside the dancing flames, that my curiosity was born.

Many more of the insights in this book have reached me through the countless words and stories of fellow travelers whom I have met on the long road of life. As I have sat by the figurative fireside, speaking with you, my family, friends, colleagues, patients, clients, and perfect strangers, you have shared your insights with me. From these gifts, I continue to stitch together the rich tapestry we call wisdom on my journey toward the truth that will always be our final destination.

I invite you to join me at the fireside. Put aside toil and ambition for a moment to engage with me in intimate conversation. Read these words with an open mind and heart.

The structure of this book reflects the way that these insights have been revealed to me, a series of lucky moments that happened upon me in no particular order. Although the individual insights have been grouped under section headers that suggest a highly organized gathering of thoughts, that grouping was, in truth, a retrospective exercise.

And so, I encourage you to explore the book in an entirely random sequence. Pick it up often. Open it to a page that catches your fancy, or to a header that resonates with you in the moment, and join me for a fireside chat on an interesting topic. As we might linger in a conversation, I hope that you will not rush through the topic. I invite you to pause and reflect; mull it over; journal to bring your thoughts to the surface; and take action. Insights that emerge without processing remain just that: insights. When you engage with them actively, they become knowledge and wisdom.

Have fun,

Roddy

INTRODUCTION

ARE YOU STANDING IN YOUR OWN WAY?

Our human brain is the pinnacle of evolution. It is our greatest gift. It also exerts astounding control over our individual and collective destinies—and it's not always helpful.

Several years ago, I published *BodyWHealth: Journey to Abundance*. Based on cutting-edge science, this first major work is a simple guide to unlocking our best possible selves. "WHealth" goes beyond just physical health and represents the potential for the full breadth of health, happiness, and prosperity that lives within each of us. Unfortunately, most of us don't enjoy these gifts to the extent we should. We are "locked" away from them by a combination of ignorance and habit. "Unlocking" them allow us to live abundantly, as Mother Nature intended.

The book presents seven keys that have been scientifically demonstrated to unlock WHealth.

BodyWHealth starts with three foundational keys for unlocking physical WHealth beyond simple health, because the body should be the starting point for every journey of self-discovery and self-actualization. In the middle of the book are two powerful keys that unlock powerful mindsets that ensure success on the journey. The book concludes with two keys that unlock emotional WHealth (that is, happiness)—the ultimate prize we all desire and deserve.

BodyWHealth was inspired by my own personal transformation.

Despite achieving substantial professional success, I was headed for personal catastrophe. I was working hard, with my eyes focused on important goals (like promotion and financial success) when I abruptly realized that I had put my most cherished assets—my health and happiness—at grave risk.

Over the period of a year, I drew on my deep scientific insight into the human condition to reboot my own life. As I tasted success, I realized for the first time that abundance is not only an attainable state but a condition for which Mother Nature has designed us…perfectly.

This phenomenon was too good to keep to myself, and so I wrote the book to share the insight I had accrued on that spectacular leg of my journey.

Since then, my journey has continued.

I have advanced my knowledge of the science of peak performance. In particular, I have deepened my insight into our brain—the ringmaster of our individual performance, or underperformance as the case may be.

Thanks to ongoing self-exploration, highly impactful work with my clients, and expanded knowledge of the rapidly evolving field of neuroscience, I now have a more profound perspective on abundance and the pathway to get there.

It is my experiences during this phase of my evolution that have inspired this new book.

Central to this new work is an alarming irony regarding the relationship we humans tend to have with our magnificent brains.

All our other organs dutifully serve our interests. When we want to go to work, we command our muscles to get us there. Our lungs dutifully breathe in and out 12 times every minute in order to deliver life-giving oxygen to our tissues and vital organs.

But, if you're brutally honest with yourself, you will acknowledge that you wake each morning to serve your brain.

If your brain says you're hungry, you head for the kitchen.

If your brain says you're sad, the day becomes gloomy.

If your brain says somebody else is trying to undermine you, you retreat into painful paranoia.

But who is this brain? And who or what authorizes it to exert so much control over your life?

You do!

Yes, each and every one of us has fallen into the trap of surrendering authority to our brains. Have you heard the expression "you're standing in your own way"? It may feel painfully familiar. More often than not, when we empower our brain as the supreme leader, our thoughts and emotions end up being a barrier to our own success. Rather than enabling us, our brain becomes an obstacle. We stand in our own way, restricting our own performance and limiting our own success.

This new book will help guide you to get out of your own way by understanding the construct of your mind and the complex cognitive, emotional, and spiritual forces that impact your happiness on the journey. It is less a detailed set of instructions based on underlying scientific facts than it is a series of colorful and practical insights and suggestions garnered from the application of this mind-blowing science in my own life and the lives of my clients (who are all referred to by different names in this work to protect their privacy).

In order to make this book highly relevant to readers, I have included a broad range of examples of how we stand in our own way. Some of these will probably come quickly to your mind: social anxiety that prevents community engagement, self-doubt that undermines the ambitious entrepreneur, and the impatience or quick temper that hampers the best efforts of a committed spouse.

Think of ways that you, your family, your friends, and your coworkers stand in your own way. Each of us delivers less than our best on most days. This is a source of immense stress and stands firmly between us and abundance.

I invite you to join me next to the warmth of the fireside of life. Engage in the conversation, with equal measures of humility and curiosity. Let's begin to understand and address this deep-rooted self-sabotage, so we can strive for abundance together. Over time, our collective wisdom will enable you to push through those self-imposed barriers to live your best life.

YOUR
MAGNIFICENT
BRAIN

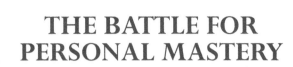

THE BATTLE FOR PERSONAL MASTERY

Despite our many differences, modern humans share a common failing: We consistently handicap our own best efforts, with disastrous consequences.

Which of the following describes you?

- *You want to be successful, but you're afraid you will fail and look stupid.*

- *You want to find a romantic partner, but you think you're too ugly.*

- *You want to be patient and kind, but you always seem to lose your temper and shout at everyone.*

- *You want to be focused on your work, but you end up wasting time on lesser priorities...or Netflix.*

- *You want to be calm, but you're always anxious.*

- *You want to welcome feedback, but you close down defensively.*

- *You want to be happy, but you wake most mornings with a head full of sadness.*

If you're anything like the rest of us, at least one of these descriptions resonates with you. Despite our different circumstances, we're all united in one common ailment: We struggle to get out of our own way.

That's right: Every one of us has a part of ourselves standing between us and success, guarding the gates of triumph.

And that part is in your head, the same place you find the greatest gift of all: your powerful brain.

Your brain is the ultimate control center. All your other organs are controlled by your brain, either consciously or subconsciously. So perhaps it's not unreasonable for the brain to assume it has responsibility beyond your physical survival.

But...

Who gave your brain permission to take over your life?

Who gave it permission to limit your happiness, your financial success, your romantic accomplishments, or the realization of your dreams?

You've probably read enough self-help articles and quotes from famous people to know who is responsible for this painful predicament. Yes, it is *you*.

We are each powerfully and individually responsible for our own limitations. We alone control our brain. We give it permission to curtail our achievements, or we license it to unlock our success.

The why and how is different for each of us. Your specific combination of hereditary traits, parental influences, and environmental pressures makes your relationship with your brain as unique as your fingerprints.

But we all have the authority to command our brains to serve our own interests and needs.

I call this *personal mastery*, because when we have all our organs, systems, and faculties working *for* us, including our brain, we have truly mastered our own biology.

Many of us spend hours, days, and even years learning to master modern technology to enhance our lives. We learn to drive cars, we employ our computers and cellphones, and we increasingly harness the collective intelligence of the Internet of Things. On top of this, we also strive to engage (or manipulate) the other humans in our biosphere for our own benefit.

Isn't it alarming that we devote so much time and effort to learning computer algorithms and digital gadgets before we have mastered our own enormous power? Isn't it strange (and even dangerous) that we're reaching beyond our own capabilities, trying to control others before we have achieved *self*-control?

Modern science has taught us that we can take clearly defined steps to achieve personal mastery. Personal mastery is achieved through knowledge of our complex neurobiology, personal insight, and hard work. Like skeletal muscles, our intellectual and emotional muscles can be trained.

Human society is advancing at a terrifying pace, much faster than the pedestrian dawdle of natural evolution. With escalating competitive pressure, life is no longer a game for amateurs.[1] One day soon, the very survival of our species, the mighty Homo sapiens, will depend on our collective personal mastery. We must each equip ourselves with the best possible insight and guidance to meet that challenge.

A VITAL PLASTIC

Ten years ago, I chose to make massive changes in my life. During that period, I stumbled across several major insights that shed new light on the way my brain was working. This knowledge transformed my life, unlocking clarity and boosting confidence in profound new ways in my personal and professional lives.

I have spent the subsequent years expanding my understanding of fundamental and applied neuroscience. There is no doubt in my mind that a single scientific finding has revolutionized our approach to unlocking our own immense potential as humans: Today, we know that we can literally reinvent ourselves by upgrading the structure and function of our (already-impressive) brains.

For many dark years, we scientists believed that the brain was a static organ. We thought that it peaked in childhood, then slowly decayed through the remaining years of our life. Today, luckily, we know better!

Our brain, the control center for our every action and the organ that separates us from all other life on this planet, is known to be highly adaptive. It is not built with cold hard-wiring like the supercomputers with which we're all increasingly familiar. Instead, it is a dynamic organ that dramatically adapts its inner working, giving you the capacity for radical transformation throughout your life.

We refer to this property as *neuroplasticity*.[2]

To clarify, the brain is not *elastic*, an organ that can stretch only to snap back into its original shape once the stretch-stimulus is ended. Instead, it is *plastic*—pliable enough for us to bend and shape, throughout our lives, to serve our current needs.

Norman Doidge, MD, describes the emergence of neuroplasticity theory in his fascinating book *The Brain That Changes Itself*.[3] There are certain important overarching principals relevant to anyone who owns a brain, such as the implications of "use it or lose it." There is such a thing as competitive plasticity and a struggle for precious real estate that happens every day within your central nervous system. It is vital to appreciate the significance of critical periods in brain development, which is why parents obsess about creating the best educational contexts for their children. There is also a science of learning and unlearning that is hugely significant in the development of good and bad habits.

Today, I work with high-performing clients from many fields. Some seek performance tweaks; others strive for radical transformation.

My coaching guides them to unlock hidden potential. In each case, I help my clients to understand optimal brain function. More importantly, we modify their beliefs, attitudes, and actions by embracing the incredible plasticity that Mother Nature has incorporated into our wondrous design.

You do not need to be the victim of a mindset cast in stone. When you can see your brain as a lump of immensely powerful clay, your future truly is in your own hands!

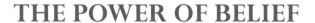

THE POWER OF BELIEF

Success is elusive, a secret understood and mastered by only a few. The good news is that success is attainable—through the power of *belief*. Belief originates deep inside your brain and can be built and developed, which means you can truly *real*-ize your own success!

In order to understand the role of our brain in belief, we need to review the evolution of this most powerful of our organs.[4]

At the center of our magnificent brain resides the most primitive part of our central nervous system. The *primitive brain* (also known as the reptilian brain) is responsible for critical survival instincts and governs fight and flight responses. It is the default brain we use at times of crisis. Driven by fear and adrenaline, this part of our brain compels us to flee from danger, to turn to meet it with aggression, or to lie low to escape detection. We need our primitive brains, but if that were all we had, we would be cold survival engines, like snakes and lizards.

Over time, early mammals added the limbic system to their primitive brains. The limbic system brings emotion and color to our world. This *emotional brain* provides a selective advantage to those species that have it because it drives us to love and nurture our offspring and to collaborate with others. The language of the emotional brain is love and empathy.

Finally, we humans added a massive cerebral cortex (the gray matter), increasing our brain to three times the size of our closest mammalian relatives. This *cognitive brain* layer introduced thought and reason, the supreme gift that clearly differentiates us from other animals. It is a powerful organ that enables us to master our environment.

These three parts of our brain are intimately connected. Millions of nerve junctions enable messages to pass between them, moderating their influence in our lives. Our overall behavior is the composite effect of the three brain centers.

In the absence of any "higher" function, the primitive brain runs wild with its negative, defensive messages that sow doubt. "Run, hide, fight!" it screams. This is useful when we are in true danger but is a highly disruptive influence the rest of the time—such as when we develop new ideas or contemplate the exciting ventures and paths that lead to success.

You see, big ideas are generated in the cognitive brain. When you generate an idea, you *want* something. When you couple it with emotion, you transform *want* into a colorful, three-dimensional *desire*, a deep and focused hunger for success.

But as we develop ideas and desires, our primitive brains are doing exactly what they have been trained to do over millions of years. Even as we picture the slim, healthy body we desire, or the castle on the hill, or the spectacular new job, or the freedom to travel, our primitive brains kick into action. They impregnate our consciousness with "protective" messages that are often disguised as simple questions:

- *What happens if I fail?*
- *What will my friends and family think of me?*
- *Why should I, who have always been unsuccessful, suddenly become wealthy?*
- *Why should the world take me seriously now?*
- *Who would even listen to my concept?*

For substantial success, you need to align your entire brain behind your idea. You need to evoke the partnership of the cognitive and emotional brains in a desire so powerful that it overrides all impedances that the primitive brain will invoke. This is belief.

Let's go back to where we started for a moment. We human beings stood out from our mammalian peers when we added a massive cerebral cortex to our brain. This gigantic leap added thought and reason to our weaponry.

The most obvious advantage to having a cognitive brain is our problem-solving ability. We are able to apply complex intellectual reasoning to address challenges and create opportunities for success. For us to take full advantage of the huge opportunity conferred on us by the cognitive layer of our brain, we need to engage it in liberating us from the restrictive doubts imposed by our primitive brain. We need to employ our cognitive powers to flood our brains with positive ideas, indirectly influencing and co-opting the emotional brain in such a way that our desires become so strong that they transform into belief.

That's when we tap into the full power of the human brain. That's when we enjoy success. That is what every highly successful person has learned to do.

The bigger the idea, the more powerfully you need to evoke the brain's pathway to belief. Once you achieve belief, success is largely inevitable. If you don't think this is true, then I invite you to study any person who has achieved grand success. Once they believed—truly *believed*—plans became actions, hopes became expectations, obstacles became challenges, and success followed.

It is important to note that achieving belief is not a linear journey, and it doesn't happen in a flash. The interactions between the three levels in the brain are more iterative, more dynamic. Belief is not an instantaneous chemical reaction. It can take time to wrestle with our primitive brain, before we finally overcome doubt with belief.

But belief is the fuel. It provides the energy, the resilience, the patience, and the strength required to get it done.

The fact that it takes time makes it harder. A moment of belief is easy. I have them all the time—often in the wee hours of the morning. But by the time I wake up to shower and dress, my trusty reptilian brain has generously offered to protect me from the pain of failure and flooded my mind with doubt.

The vast majority of us wrestle every day with doubt. On some days, we enable belief to get the upper hand and drive success, while on other days we live under the defensive cloud of our primitive brains. You may have to work actively to uphold your belief for a long time in order to deliver success.

But, if we understand the roles of the three layers in our human brain and the relationships between them, and we fully appreciate the evolutionary power of the cognitive brain, and we closely observe highly successful people, we should be filled with optimism.

So, how do you train your brain to believe? Here are some suggestions:

- *Understand and accept the voice of your primitive brain without legitimizing it.* This is a critically important nuance to your overall success. You have now learned about the existence of your primitive brain and understand that it is an important part of who you are. It protects you from catastrophe. Respect it. Understand its role. Accept that it will (and should) always have an opinion. But *do not* give it too much attention. It is much like a whiny child. You have to take heed of it. Take a quick look to see that there is no major disaster that you have overlooked, and then ignore it. Attention reinforces its bad behavior. Distract and, if necessary, overwhelm it with positive thoughts.

- *Do first the things you're avoiding most.* If you're unsure where the voice of doubt is hurting you most, pull out your to-do list. Look at those items that slide from day to day. They're often the most important tasks. The things you dread bring you closest to your inner doubt, face to face with your reptilian brain. It's understandable that you want to stay away from this monster, but don't give it the upper hand. We often overestimate the time required for unpalatable tasks, justifying that we'll get to them when we have the time. Turn them into ten-minute challenges. You'll be surprised how many of them start to disappear with a few minutes of concerted effort.

- *Think positively.* This sounds so easy, doesn't it? Scientists call this *autosuggestion*.[5] We know that we control the cognitive brain. We know that the cognitive brain influences the emotional brain and is able to override the primitive brain. Use it. Flood your brain with positive statements about your inevitable success. Repeat them over and over again. We know that the cognitive brain is highly susceptible to suggestion; use this property to ensure that your cognitive brain is teeming with positive thoughts. If your reptilian brain can seize the autopilot and drive you toward failure, then you can just as easily grab the controls and drive toward success.

- *Empathize with your idea.* Olympic champions do this when they practice visualization.[6] They spend long hours building the complete image of success in their minds, using all their senses. Spend time building the mental image of success until you can see, hear, taste, smell, and feel it vividly in your mind.

- *Repeat.* Your positive rhetoric must be a daily habit. Write your success statement down. Learn it by heart. Say it out loud throughout the day. Turn it into a song and sing it. Paste it on the wall, the roof, or the steering wheel of your car. Keep it alive.

- *Surround yourself with positive people.* If you don't have them, search for them, find them, and embrace them. Every positive echo to your positive thoughts is like gold. "Can-do" is infectious.

- *Avoid negative people.* In fact, run from them—as fast as you can. The voice of your primitive brain is loud enough. You don't need a team of naysayers augmenting these undermining pulls.

- *Fake it to make it.* In the early stages, you might have a desire that is not quite ready to be a belief. That's okay, but keep the struggle internal. On the outside, project the success that you desire. I don't suggest in any way that you become insincere. Rather, the act of designing, building, and maintaining your "game face" is a powerful, reinforcing cognitive discipline.

- *Practice.* For most of us, this habit is new or underdeveloped. Practice on the small things every day.

- *Stand tall.* Practice victory. Seriously, stand the way you will when you achieve the success you desire. Raise your arms into a **V** for victory. Your brain listens to your body. (You'll read more about this later.) These physical messages become imprinted in your thoughts and actions. You can posture your way to your goals.

- *Move along the action word list.* Success is no accident; it's a deliberate journey. Track your progress actively. Make sure that you move from *imagine* to *want* to *desire* to *believe* to *plan* to *act* to *expect* to *demand* to *anticipate* and finally, to *celebrate* success. You may move back and forward along this continuum, and that's okay. Write down where you are today, and use the power of your cognitive brain to ensure that your entire being moves toward success.

Look around you. Only a tiny minority are hugely successful in any sphere of human performance. Sadly, most people believe that they are already doing and being their best and that success is a reward for only a lucky few. They are wrong. Success is attainable through the power of belief, and belief can be nurtured. This puts your success within reach; it truly is in your power to grab it.

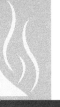

STAND TALL TO SUCCEED

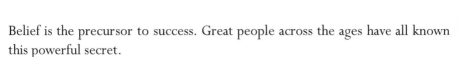

Belief is the precursor to success. Great people across the ages have all known this powerful secret.

Each one of us has the right to achieve success in our lives and the ability to learn to believe. Here is one simple way to engage your body to launch you toward success.

Early in our development, we learn to read body language. Even before we can understand spoken language, we react to the touch and gestures of our parents and families. Deep inside, our brains are constantly observing and reacting to non-verbal cues from the people we interact with.[7]

But what about our own body language? How does our brain react to this?

Picture a low point in your life. Visualize yourself when you were filled with doubt and fear. See yourself in detail in the theatre of your mind. What do you see? You were small, hunched, and closed. Your voice and non-verbal gestures were small. You shuffled along with cautious, little steps.

Now transport yourself to a moment of success, a triumphal event when your mind was filled with elation and pride. Again, picture yourself. How did you appear to the world? You stood tall and open. Your head was high and your shoulders back. You may even have raised both arms above your head in the broad **V** for victory. Your stride was long and meaningful. Your voice was strong and your gestures generous.

We know that our bodies mirror our feelings. When we are afraid, our bodies shrink away from the world. When we are successful, our bodies expand and stand tall with pride. Our body language is highly responsive to our emotional state.

But what about the reverse? Does our brain listen to our body language?

Science is beginning to answer this question for us, and the conclusions are robust. Here is the exciting truth: Our brains watch our body language and learn from it. When we act powerless, we become powerless.

But, when we act powerful, we become powerful!

Researchers have shown how we are able to change our mindset by changing our posture.[8] It all started with a smile. Many years ago, social scientists asked people to put a pencil into their mouths, holding it horizontally between their lips in a manner that forced a smile. Nothing else changed except that their facial gesture was forced into a fake smile…and they became happy.

A lot more research has been done since then to not only prove the science but also demonstrate the mechanism. Two critical hormones mediate the balance of confidence we enjoy in our lives. Testosterone is the hormone of positivity and power (both men and women have it, but at different concentrations). Cortisol is the stress hormone of negativity and doubt. Powerful, successful people tend to have higher levels of testosterone and lower levels of cortisol.[9]

Here is the liberating science: If you adopt a power pose for as little as two minutes, you increase your levels of testosterone and decrease your levels of cortisol.[10] Your brain senses these changes, and your level of self-belief rises. Researchers have demonstrated in several different situations how this simple act not only improves your own belief but spills out to influence those around you. When you believe and they believe, success flows for everyone!

Amy Cuddy, a social scientist from Harvard, recommends a simple daily ritual: Stand tall with an open body in an explicit power pose for two minutes every day.[11] Allow your brain to enjoy the boost of testosterone and reduced levels of cortisol. Do this before important meetings, sporting events, or performances, and your elevated self-confidence will translate into enhanced performance.

For many years, personal coaches have advocated that their clients fake it until they make it. We have now substantiated the science behind this advice. We now know that our bodies can change our minds. You *can* fake it until you believe it. And then…

When you believe it, you *will* make it.

PROMOTING POSITIVITY

Have you ever noticed that your focus shifts when you're preparing to make an important decision? Let's take buying a new car as an example. Whereas on any other day I get into my car and drive to a meeting with my attention on the natural beauty or people around me, life is very different when I'm getting ready to buy a car. Until the purchase is complete, all I see are the other vehicles on the road. "Ooh, that's a nice one, perhaps I should look at that make." Or, "Wow, that's a beautiful color; I should get one of those." The natural and human beauty that surrounds me and the music on the radio get completely overwhelmed by auto obsession.

I'm sure that you've experienced something similar when buying cars, or cameras, or phones, or choosing a college, or even choosing a mate. Your brain focuses in on your obsession, minimizing all other stimuli.

There's a simple, biological reason for this phenomenon. It's an ingenious neurological gift from Mother Nature designed to improve our survival and success.

But heed this warning: It can also be our downfall.

You see, as our brains evolved, Mother Nature gave us spectacular computing capabilities to process incoming data. This tremendous neurological capacity created a new challenge: data overload. Scientists estimate that we have to process several million data points at any one moment, and the neuroscientists at the Laboratory of Neuro Imaging at the University of Southern California estimate that we have between 60,000 and 70,000 thoughts in a day.[12] That's more than 4,000 thoughts per hour, more than 60 thoughts per minute, and more than one thought per second. That's a lot to process!

Picture yourself in a massive airport or train station or market, and you can imagine the problem our powerful brains have on an ongoing basis: noise, noise, noise.

Mother Nature designed a remarkable filtering system to help us manage this flood of incoming data. This function is housed in a collection of neurological centers that are known as the Reticular Activating System (RAS).[13] The RAS is clustered near the entrance to our magnificent brain and works a bit like the switch system at a large train station, channeling, filtering, and integrating the sensory messages that come into our brains. The RAS also plays a similar role in processing outgoing messages from our emotional and cognitive brains.

The primary role of the RAS is actually in moderating our levels of alertness, so it is intimately involved with regulating sleep and wakefulness.[14] But it also has this more delicate influence on our attention and focus. The RAS is the filter that sifts through the millions of incoming signals that arrive in your brain every second, enabling you to process your environment without your head exploding.[15] The RAS decides what we *actually* hear and see, effectively reducing the noise to a small group of stimuli that we can handle while filtering out millions of "distractions."

You can probably see how this system enhanced our survival in the wild, and anybody who has been in a life-threatening emergency will verify this. When our ancestors were fleeing from a charging wooly mammoth, their brains were keenly focused on their escape route, ignoring the delicate beauty and fragrance of the flowers they trampled in their hasty retreat. Similarly, when I'm preoccupied with choosing a new car, all I can see after stepping out of my front door are cars, cars, and more cars.

There is a powerful beauty in this system that we can harness for health and happiness. But there is an equally powerful danger we must avoid. The secret to this power lies in the override of the cognitive and emotional brains. You see, it's the higher centers in our brain that tell the RAS what is important—whether positive or negative.[16] Your RAS listens carefully to the thoughts bouncing around in your cognitive brain and draws its conclusions about their importance to you. It determines that the thoughts you have most frequently are the important ones, and then it performs its single-minded (pardon the pun) duty of *perceptual integration*.[17]

Let's look at two different scenarios to understand the far-reaching implications of this elegant system.

Have you ever noticed how powerful your negative thoughts are? That's because you reinforce them with the help of your RAS. Have you ever heard your own voice in your head saying, "Life is tough," or "I'm not smart," or "I can't make anybody happy," or "I don't deserve to be healthy, or happy, or prosperous"? Well, the first place that registers these statements is your RAS. It takes careful note of these powerful seeding thoughts and then starts to select for those incoming messages that reinforce that belief…simply because you told it to. So, you selectively begin to notice that life is hard, or that you're not smart. Your RAS effectively shows you the things that prove this belief to be true while minimizing all evidence to the contrary. And soon, your initial statement becomes a deeply held belief, reinforced by the "facts" your RAS presents to you.

I hope that you see how flawed and dangerous this can be. The good news is that you can instead choose to embrace the other end of the spectrum of possibilities. Have you ever heard your voice in your head saying, "Life is beautiful," or "I'm always lucky," or "I have a gift to make people happy," or "I deserve health, and happiness, and prosperity"? When you choose to utter the positive instead of the negative, your RAS responds dutifully, focusing your attention on those data points that prove the truth in your statement while minimizing data that may dispute it, reinforcing your initial positive thoughts.

This is why gratitude is so powerful. Because your cognitive brain is under your complete voluntary control, you decide what messages bounce around inside of it. As you articulate the list of items for which you are grateful, your RAS is eavesdropping. It gets to work and finds abundant proof that reinforces your appreciation. If you're thankful for love, you'll be bathed in love. If you're appreciative of health, you'll experience good health. If you're grateful for friendship, you'll be surrounded by friends. If you decide that you will fill your brain with positive thoughts, your loyal RAS will filter through positive data from the outside, reinforcing the positive melody in your mind. Life will look better, sound better, and feel better—and with this uplifting feedback, you will be in a more powerful position to live your life and deliver on your dreams.

The powerful gifts of positive thinking and gratitude can transform your life by unlocking the power of your RAS. Practice them consciously, introducing them into your daily routine. Start today, and remember that habits take seven weeks to become established. Use a piece of paper, a journal, or an app to capture both positive thoughts and gratitude meticulously for those seven weeks. Your RAS will watch, filter, and integrate—and then you can watch your life transform for the better.

I'll leave you with this compelling poem. The author is unknown, though you'll find it attributed to many great leaders.[18] In the absence of definite ownership, I choose to allocate it to Mother Nature, who designed this wondrous system in the first place:

Watch your thoughts, for they become words.

Watch your words, for they become actions.

Watch your actions, for they become habits.

Watch your habits, for they become your character.

And watch your character, for it becomes your destiny.

THE MAGIC OF
IMAGINATION

*"Imagination is more important than knowledge.
For knowledge is limited to all we now know and understand,
while imagination embraces the entire world,
and all there ever will be to know and understand."*

~ Albert Einstein

*Growing up in South Africa, I often sat watching lion cubs in
the wild. If you've had this privilege, I'm sure that you too were
mesmerized by their miniature worlds. They start as cute little
balls of fluff that you want to hold and cuddle, and they end up
as majestic killers. How is this massive transformation possible?
Of course, there is something in their DNA that drives a biological
maturation process, but there is more to this mystery.*

*The clue is in watching the play of these furry cubs as they begin
to explore their world.*

*These little creatures engage in robust physical play. They stalk,
pounce, chew, bite, ambush, and chase each other continuously.
Their comical antics are punctuated only by periods of feeding
and sleep. In their little minds, the flicking tail of their mother
becomes the prey that will feed their own offspring. As they stalk
their sister, they imagine a juicy fat antelope. As they square up
against their brother, bristling and snarling, standing as tall as
possible, they imagine themselves defending their pride against
competing predators.*

These imaginary games empower their future.

To understand this, we must understand the neurobiology of the brain. A powerful
thought or idea that originates in the cerebral cortex, when coupled with a strong
desire from the emotional brain, becomes belief, which in turn suppresses the
negative, protective influence of the primitive brain. Belief is the cornerstone of
the mansion of success.

That's why lion cubs play. They are exercising their brains in the aspiration and idea of future success.[19]

That's why children play, too.

What did you pretend to be when you were growing up? A doctor, a nurse, an astronaut, a soldier, a teacher, a dolphin trainer? In playing these imaginary games, you were planting some of the most important seeds of your life. If you carefully peel back the layers of memory, you will realize that you weren't pretending to be a cowboy, but rather that, in your mind, you actually *were* one. You weren't pretending to be a caring teacher educating and nurturing little human beings; you actually *were* one.

This is the power of imagination.

But these games aren't only for cubs and kids. They are the foundation of success for adults, too.

Walt Disney could not have built his fantastical entertainment empire without imagination. Steve Jobs could not have built the Apple technological powerhouse without first imagining beautiful, sleek devices that would one day connect us intimately with those we love. We would not have put Neil Armstrong on the moon if not for the powerful imagination of early NASA scientists.

Every journey starts with a vision, a tiny seed from your cognitive brain that grows in your imagination. Nurtured by desire from your emotional brain, it becomes belief and fuels success.

Plant seeds. Play. Imagine. Dream. Believe!

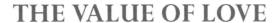

THE VALUE OF LOVE

I spend my days working with senior business leaders—CEOs who are determined to bring their very best into their roles as organizational leaders.

Much of my work focuses on the cognitive brain: the massive cerebral cortex that hosts the faculties of thought and reason. Only when we understand the potential of the cognitive brain can we contemplate success. The end point of this mastery is a profound state of self-belief. When we attain this, we invite prosperity in its broadest possible interpretation.

Most of my executive clients would be satisfied to stop here, but I always urge them to journey further in search of even deeper personal power. You see, Mother Nature gave us another major gift, also housed within our complex brain, one that we seldom think about in the context of our professional aspirations. When we understand the science of our emotional brain, we can unlock the power of love, with very tangible benefits both at work and at home.

Before we explore these synergistic endowments, let's contemplate the lives of reptiles, who lack both of these brain parts and their associated benefits.

Snakes and lizards are cold-blooded creatures with tiny heads. Mother Nature programmed their primitive reptilian brains with instincts for fight and flight— and not much else. Reptiles give birth to huge numbers of tiny babies, hoping desperately that a few will survive. Hundreds, even thousands, die before reaching adulthood. Those that are lucky enough to survive to adulthood live isolated lives, surviving on their individual skills.

These creatures are programed to stay away from others to survive; by design, they are ruled by fear and suspicion.

That same reptilian brain is alive and well deep inside of our advanced human brains. It's our default mode in times of stress. You know the feelings well; if you're anxious, scared, or angry, your primitive reptilian brain is hard at work. That's okay for short bursts of survival-related activity, but when prolonged, it has disastrous consequences for your health and happiness.

That is where the emotional brain comes into play, with its capacity for affection. To connect our emotional brain with the rest of the body—linking the command center with the arms, legs, and organs that would act out loving behaviors—Mother Nature constructed two biological bridges: one chemical, using hormones that spread through the bloodstream to distant sites, and the other electrical, using a system of nerves specifically designed for non-urgent signaling.

Hormones are particular kinds of chemicals—proteins, actually—that are produced by specialized glands and secreted into the bloodstream. Once in the blood, they circulate throughout the body. Certain tissues and organs have receptors designed for these chemical messengers, inducing very specific actions at the target sites. It's an effective way to diffuse custom signals deep into our body.

One of the emotion-related hormones is *oxytocin*.[20] It induces a range of positive feelings, such as affection, trust, and empathy, while reducing fear and anxiety. These benefits allow us to enjoy social proximity with others, leading to the colloquial name for this powerful chemical: the "love hormone." More than this, oxytocin is intimately involved in procreation—in bonding, birthing, and nursing.

Mother Nature didn't stop there. She also empowered oxytocin with some very important responsibilities with significant impact on our overall health. This magical hormone also suppresses levels of pro-inflammatory cytokines, the chemical messengers that promote degeneration and decay.[21] By moderating the fire of inflammation, oxytocin promotes healing and regeneration—two critical elements of well-being. That's right: Love and the act of loving fight degeneration and decay, making us not only happy but healthy, too!

The second enhancement designed to bridge our emotional brains with our obedient bodies was an upgrade to our nervous system. You remember the nerves of fear that travel through the spinal cord to the body? They are collectively known as the *sympathetic nervous system* and enable flight and fight.

The upgrade introduced an opposing wiring known as the *parasympathetic nervous system* that carries messages to invoke relaxation along a giant chemical pathway known as the *vagus nerve*.

The vagus nerve slows us down. Under its command, our gastrointestinal system stocks up on vital energy and nutrients, and the cells of regeneration and repair get to work restoring our vital tissues.[22] This physical state takes us off the high alert induced by the sympathetic nervous system, thus favoring social connectivity.

The vagal override that takes place only in mammals has recently revealed even deeper benefits, including profound changes in the activity of genes that regulate inflammation and immunity.[23] Feelings of deep emotional well-being (known as *eudemonic well-being* to distinguish it from a more superficial feeling of satisfaction, known as *hedonic well-being*) activate genes that promote healing, recovery, and a healthy immune system and switch off genes that promote disease-causing inflammation and degeneration.

The overt purpose is simple: When we're in danger, we may need inflammatory cells to cope with acute injury, and we can't waste energy in long-term restorative processes. But, when there is no danger, under the influence of the vagus nerve, our bodies get to work fighting cancer, preventing degeneration, and restoring healthy tissue in vital organs like the heart and brain.

Why is this complex science important to busy, results-driven CEOs?

It's simple. The adrenaline- and fear-based drivers of performance are excellent in stimulating survival and short bursts of high performance. And self-belief driven by cognitive competence remains the pillar of human performance. But *enduring* success requires that we regenerate vital resources and reserves at least as much as we consume and destroy them. We neglect the role of the emotional brain and that critical vagus nerve at our peril.

So, my overall guidance to leaders who aspire to long-term success includes this surprising advice:

- Breathe deeply. Deep breathing, especially with the prolonged exhalation that is a common meditative practice, stimulates the vagus nerve.[24]

- Get down on your knees and pray, or if you don't want to pray, then get down on the floor and do yoga, stretch, or meditate. Self-effacing, respectful postures like bending, bowing, and kneeling all stimulate pressure receptors in the vagus nerve, inducing its downstream benefits.[25]

- Sing out loud. Singing, chanting, and praying out loud are all common elements of many religions—probably because their early practitioners discovered empirically that all those activities stimulate the vagus nerve![26]

- Play a musical instrument, especially a brass or wind instrument.

- And, love without restraint!

When you get this right, you won't only *do* better; you will also *feel* better. More importantly, you will *be* better; you will substantially reduce your risk of devastating disease and premature death. In doing so, you avail yourself of the full package: professional success, health, happiness, and longevity. It's a no-brainer!

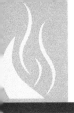

A NATURAL UPGRADE
FOR YOUR BRAIN

In the shadow of the great pandemic of the 21st century, there has been a massive swing away from working in the office in favor of working from home—or almost anywhere, really. I believe that one of the factors driving this new employee-driven workplace trend is the recognition that our environment is an integral part of our professional performance, a truth strongly supported by emerging brain science.[27]

As an executive coach, I ensure that each of the highly successful senior leaders with whom I work understands and respects our universal context: that we are natural beings, created within natural laws and a natural world. We forget this at our peril.

Three major principles underpin our relationship with nature:

1. *When we understand our evolutionary context and our natural design, we can easily determine the right things to do for our body. It's an ingenious design, where the incentive and the reward are the same: health and happiness.*

2. *We are natural beings, integrated into a vast ecosystem of animals, vegetables, and minerals. When we attempt to isolate ourselves from this system, we put our physical, emotional, and mental well-being at substantial risk.*

3. *The human brain is our greatest asset, differentiating us from all other life forms. This critical organ is at the center of our relationship with our environment and plays a massive role in our health and happiness.*

Today, we have increasing scientific evidence demonstrating the benefits of nature for our mental and emotional health. The value of *green space* (sometimes dubbed "Vitamin G") and *blue space* (ranging from massive oceans to tiny ponds and office water features) has been documented in great detail.[28] Many invisible chemicals and aromas (known as *phytoncides*) have delicate benefits on our cognitive and emotional functioning.[29] Aromatherapy, gardening and "wilderness therapy," pet ownership, and "brain food" are among the many therapeutic approaches being researched today that harness the power of nature for our benefit.

So, what do we do to capitalize on the vast body of emerging evidence that green spaces, blue spaces, and every natural environment in between is good for us?

Go to nature. We should be outside more. We should be taking advantage of "green exercise." Many of us have moved away from constrained indoor exercise spaces, perhaps initially forced to by the 2020 pandemic shutdowns and later choosing to because of newly discovered preference. Frankly, whatever the reason, I sincerely hope that you exercise outside from now on—it's so much better for your mind and body.

And while you're at it, why not work outside? A brisk walk through nature as you talk to a colleague or listening to the birds chirp as you sit on a bench with your laptop will increase your mental clarity and productivity. Or you could compose emails under the spreading canopy of your favorite tree. Or practice your next big presentation with the squirrels and the birds as your audience.

Why not eat meals outside, too? You can please all your senses and find great tranquility by savoring your food in the great outdoors.

Bring nature to you. Put green and blue features into your home and office. Ask office managers to build a courtyard for your workplace. Petition city planners to spend your tax dollars on natural features in your town or city. Vote for leaders who support these uplifting initiatives.

And if they won't, stay home! Yes, stay home, and tell them why. Tell them that not only can you get more work done at home but you can take a walk outside between meetings in your carefully nurtured green space. You can more easily maintain your physical health, you'll be more emotionally resilient, and your mental productivity will go up noticeably.

That should make *them* happy…and, even better, you!

(If you're looking for a thorough overview of our current scientific knowledge on the impact of the natural environment on our human brains, you may enjoy Eva Selhub and Alan Logan's book *Your Brain on Nature.*[30])

A VALUABLE LIFE LESSON FROM A TINY FEATHERED FRIEND

I live in a house with big sliding glass doors that invite fresh air to wash freely through the home.

With doors that are left wide open, I often have unexpected feathered visitors. They dart into the house, not noticing that they are leaving the leafy garden to enter a modern brick construction.

I'm usually alerted to their entrance by the excited barking of my little dog, driven as much by curiosity as by instinct. The lounge erupts into chaos, with Skittles leaping and lunging after the frightened bird. The little creature flaps hopelessly from wall to ceiling, leaving a trail of feathers behind.

When this happens, I work to calm down both the delicate little visitor and the excited dog before quietly shepherding the bird toward an open door to escape back to the great outdoors.

But one day—one bird—was different.

Although the bird was trapped inside, he was calm.

He sat on the back of a chair, his head cocked to one side, and looked at me with an air of intrigue. Almost reluctantly, I steered him toward the open door. He settled confidently on the railing of the wooden deck outside.

We held each other's gaze for a while. In that tranquil moment, I realized that this little bird was a great teacher.

From time to time, we human beings become trapped on our journeys. We find ourselves in unfamiliar places, seemingly ensnared by the vagaries of life.

As happens with most of the birds that have come into my house, fear and panic incapacitate us. Without clarity of thought, we fly around desperately, crashing into walls and hiding in dark corners.

What we don't realize is that we are incapacitated by *our own thoughts*. There are always solutions to our most pressing problems, just as the wide-open doors of my house offer a solution to the trapped birds. But panic makes us blind to them.

Mother Nature has given humans the immense gift of our prefrontal cortex. With practice, we learn to operate from this powerful part of our brain in a state of mindfulness. This most recently evolved area in our brain serves as a refuge from the chaos of our own neurobiology—a place where we escape helplessness, calmly aware of our own thoughts and emotions.

Mindfulness helps us to stay calm when the world erupts into chaos around us. And, like my little feathered friend, when we're calm, we find solutions for life's most difficult challenges.

Instead of panic, we enjoy peace and liberation.

I hope that you too will meet little emissaries from Mother Nature on your journey. Even more, I hope that you will explore the power of mindfulness and will learn to exploit the intense calm of the present moment in your own beautiful life.

RELATIONSHIP
WITH SELF

THE NATURE OF PERSONAL GROWTH

Mary was in tears. She had come to me in desperation.

You wouldn't know that she was in trouble to look at her, because outwardly she was joyful and kind. Her friends and colleagues didn't know she was desperate, because she was a loyal companion and recognized as one of the most generous mentors at work. Even her loving husband didn't realize the extent of her torment, because she worked hardest to keep things together at home.

Not so inside…

Inside, she felt overwhelmed. She felt she was always rushing, under-serving all her important people. The coping mechanisms she'd developed over a lifetime of success seemed to be failing her. She was afraid that she was disappointing at home and at work, despite ample evidence to the contrary.

These should have been years of celebration for her, a phase of joy and ease. Her children were grown, successfully launched on their own independent journeys. She had a strong reputation in the local business community and beyond.

Yet, she was desperate. Despite looking happy, she really didn't feel it.

Halfway through our discussion, she used the phrase that I have heard so often when good people lose their way:

"Roddy, I'm just so tired of wearing the mask."

Of course, she was not referring to the physical masks we wore to protect one another from potentially deadly illness during the great pandemic that changed the world in 2020. Wearing those life-saving masks was a gift we gave one another.

It is the metaphorical masks that so many of us wear behind the physical ones that are the problem. They are one of life's fundamental challenges, and here is the reason:

We are, at our very core, natural beings. Like all living beings, we are dynamic—both physically and psychically.

Our psychic destiny is growth. And when we grow, when we expand our consciousness, we are happy.

But you can't grow inside the rigid form of a metaphorical mask.

Perhaps for a time, often as young adults, we grow to fill our metaphorical mask. Having decided to be a physician, or a businessperson, or an artist, or an international athlete, we know what it takes. And so, we build ourselves out within that mask to fulfill our dreams. We fake it until we make it. And many of us are successful in doing so.

For a time, we are happy—even if we're not entirely comfortable with the fact that the mask has been largely designed by society's expectations of us rather than by our own desires.

But then, sooner or later, the pain of stasis starts eroding our well-being.

Too many people then freeze, too frightened or embarrassed to drop the mask. They fear that introspection will destroy the (false) happiness they have built. They are terrified that they will look unsuccessful in front of family, friends, and colleagues. They are afraid that a courageous pause to reevaluate their purpose and direction will end in a disastrous downward spiral.

These people hide from their pain in many ways. It may be alcohol, or drugs, or other abusive manifestations. Often, it's simply overwork. They hide behind a fierce wall of determination, pretending that the world simply wouldn't survive without them and continuing in their unhappiness.

But the bold few who dive into self-examination are rewarded.

They ask the big questions and find the big answers. Growth is their reward, and happiness is the currency of that reward.

Think of how relieved we felt when, as the pandemic subsided, we could safely remove our physical masks after months of wearing them, showing each other our full faces again. That same relief is waiting for you when you dare to remove your metaphorical mask and explore the true self waiting beneath.

Like you, Mary is a beautiful, hard-working, powerful being. She has now started a new growth spurt. She's excited (and a little nervous), and I am honored to be her guide. She will unlock many riches on this next phase of her journey.

What about you? When your next growth spurt arrives, what will you do?

IN SEARCH OF SELF

There is one tiny, three-word question that can evoke a flood of confusion and pain or offer us the potential to unlock a life of well-earned peace and joy. It is, in fact, the ultimate existential question.

Who am I?

If you're a warm-blooded, thinking human being, you too have been challenged by this perplexing topic.

I spent many hours reflecting on this as a young man, without ever really finding resolution. Today, I answer the question with some confidence. I'm not sure that I have the final answer, and like any good scientist I'm open to being entirely wrong.

But I believe that each of us has two intimately intertwined and interdependent selves.

The first I refer to as the "authentic SELF." It's the *you* that is there at the very beginning, and the *you* that is there throughout your life. The enormity of the mystery of this personhood is well beyond our current scientific insights, but it's my personal belief that a divine superpower creates this unique and special SELF.

When you see this SELF as divinely made, it's easy to appreciate that our fundamental essence (perhaps it's our soul) has been made with boundless love, no garbage included. This is the joyful, curious, creative, confident spirit that shines undiluted in children. It is the uncontaminated simplicity and optimism of youth.

The other self is man-made…or, more accurately, mind-made.

As you know, we humans have been gifted with a massively powerful brain, which is traditionally viewed as the seat of our consciousness. It plays a highly significant role in who we are. And of course, the most primal of that brain's functions, the one it defaults to even without conscious thought, is to keep us safe.

This protective-above-all neurobiology is active throughout our life, especially when we're young and vulnerable. During these critical formative years, our brain responds and evolves to protect us from real and perceived threats. The result is the secondary and reactive mind-made self, which dilutes the authentic SELF as it forms.

The problem is that our cerebral real estate is limited; our brain physically cannot grow or expand due to our hard, bony skulls. So, the emergence of the mind-made self comes at the expense of the original, authentic SELF.

As proposed in a range of scientific models by such brain experts as Freud, Jung, Gestalt, Schwarts, Goulding, and others, we reach adulthood with a complicated psychic design composed of protective mind-made parts huddled around—and sometimes obscuring—the quintessential, authentic SELF.

Given the complexity of our personality mosaic, it's not surprising that so many of us end up struggling with that weighty existential question, "Who am I?"

The truth is that we are both of those selves. We are a colorful, dynamic montage that shifts situationally in order to survive.

But this complex design can cause us profound distress.

The workings of the mind-made self are often contrary to the instincts of the authentic SELF. For example, our primitive, child-like SELF wants to trust others, while our mind-made adult self, having experienced the pain of disappointment, arms us with the shield of suspicion and the sword of mistrust.

These intrinsic tensions drive our everyday psychic pain. The power struggle between our protective neurobiology, which is based in fear, and our fundamental essence, which is characterized by positivity and love, undermines our happiness and robs us of our peace.

When we understand this to be a potent source of our prevailing anxiety, restlessness, and discontent, the road ahead becomes clear. It is immensely valuable to identify who we truly are—to differentiate between the authentic SELF and the mind-made self and to moderate the extent to which the latter governs our thoughts and emotions.

When we limit the intrusion of the mind-made self, we get out of our own way, freeing our authentic SELF to lead us down the road to peace and happiness.

TAKING CARE OF
YOUR SELF

My client John was obviously anxious. "I'm not used to being the one who needs help," he blurted out, even before we could start formal introductions.

Through our early coaching sessions, he told me his story.

John was a professional, a fellow physician. He was exhausted. From the day he left high school, he had been on a mission. He cared deeply about people and wanted to help those suffering under the burden of disease. He had given of himself, unselfishly, throughout his exceptional career.

But now, he was burned out, with nothing more to give.

Life is a delicate balance between taking care of yourself and taking care of others. An error in either direction can have a serious negative impact on your health and happiness.

Gratitude is a powerful healing force that I recommend to all my clients. Early on, I give them a homework assignment designed to find and celebrate their strengths.

If you'd asked me to do this for John, it would've taken me less than five minutes. I could have come up with a thorough inventory of wonderful assets: intelligence, sensitivity, empathy, compassion, kindness, strength, an analytical mind, foresight… and the list would have continued.

But John really struggled with the task.

As he worked through his homework, the shocking reality dawned on him: He was almost invisible to himself.

Through years of service to others, he had carefully directed his full attention away from himself.

Lucky patients. Lucky colleagues. Lucky spouse. Lucky children.

Unlucky John!

Over several months, with deep reflection and courageous honesty, we revealed the underlying reasons for his habitual self-sacrifice and we rediscovered his appreciation for his innate value.

Today, John will share his strengths with you with appropriate modesty, but real pride. He still appreciates the benefits of purposeful living, serving a cause bigger than himself. But he now understands that this is only possible when complemented by adequate self-care.

I have met too many invisible people, especially in humanitarian professions, who hide from their inner fears in outward service to others. The outcome, while initially beautiful, is not enduring.

Unreplenished giving is simply not sustainable.

Like you, John is a hard-working, caring human being. He had the courage to reach out for help and, more importantly, to undertake an inner pilgrimage. His bravery has been rewarded, and he is now more fully alive again, excited about his future.

What about you? How good are you at taking care of yourself?

Here is a simple test for you: Do you find it easy to come up with birthday or holiday gift ideas for family members but struggle to give them a list of ideas for yourself?

If so, perhaps it's time for your own inner journey. These three steps will get you started:

1. Write down a list of your strengths.

2. Transform these words into gratitude statements that identify the value of each strength to you and to others.

3. Read the gratitude statements out loud, every day. Write them on your calendar; place sticky notes that capture them in prominent places in your home and at work. Share them with others.

You are designed for success—and taking care of yourself is an excellent place to start!

UNSTOPPABLE YOU

My role as exercise scientist and sport physician was to prepare elite athletes to win Olympic medals. I was responsible for bringing them the best science to guide their preparation and competition. We performed extensive testing on each athlete on a regular basis in our high-performance laboratory. Many of the tests were designed to take the individual to complete exhaustion as we sought to define and then shift their limits.

One afternoon, I put an elite rower through the most stringent of physiological tests. I only stopped when she was at the point of complete exhaustion. As we terminated the test, she ripped off the face mask that was measuring her oxygen consumption and let out a massive roar that shook the sides of the building before collapsing on the floor next to the ergometer.

Brigitte was a gold medalist in three consecutive Olympic Games, and she had just demonstrated why. When she should have had no more physical reserves, she was able to muster enough mental and emotional energy to let out this triumphant roar.

She was unstoppable.

Can you remember a time when you were unstoppable?

There have been several moments in my life when I felt truly unstoppable: the day I got married, the day I was awarded my medical degree, and several memorable athletic victories where it seemed that I could do nothing wrong. I was simply unstoppable.

When I worked with Olympic athletes, I became fascinated by the subtle differences between them that made one a champion and another simply a contender.

My experience with Brigitte started my lifelong quest to capture and share the science behind the unstoppable state.

Like me, I'm sure you feel frustrated at the number of times that you underperform. Even when we know we could do better, we somehow seem to get in our own way, limiting our own performance.

Fortunately, as seen throughout this book, the science of being unstoppable is beginning to emerge.

By applying modern neuroscience and established scientific approaches for achieving mastery over our thoughts, I have devised a methodology that systematically guides my clients to achieve this elusive state.

We are designed to be successful. Mother Nature has gifted us all with the capacity to be unstoppable.

But in reality, most of us subconsciously limit our own performance using intrinsic neuro-protective mechanisms that are designed to ensure our survival.

Survival was, of course, the earliest goal. But we have evolved beyond this endpoint. Today, we strive for far more. Our definition of success is far grander.

In her wisdom, Mother Nature has hardwired us with the capacity to override these powerful but limiting protective systems. Understanding this science enables us to unlock peak performance in a systematic, reliable, and repeatable manner.

More than ever before, we are able to determine our own futures. Success is in our own hands...if we only choose to grab it.

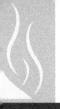

HARNESSING THE BIOLOGY OF REWARD

How many times have you tried to lose weight, get fit, stop procrastinating, or stop drinking? Think back to the many times throughout your life that you tried to make a big change. Did it work?

I bet that, as you read this, you will reflect with great sadness on many unsuccessful attempts to do something that you really wanted to do. I'm sure that you can still feel the bitter aftertaste of failure.

And what happened when you failed? When you tried to lose weight but plunged your hand into the cookie jar on the ninth day of your diet? You felt totally miserable, right? And then you ate some more to try to heal the pain of failure. And before you knew it, you had spiraled out of control, and you had a million excuses for why you'd try again next Monday, or next month, or maybe even next year. But none of those excuses made you feel any better. You just felt downright miserable!

Our best efforts are often sabotaged by a mindset that sets us up for failure, especially if we're high achievers. And it's counterintuitive, because we generally regard this specific mindset as a great asset. In fact, I'm sure that you deliberately teach your children to embrace this mindset, because we live in a culture where winning is cherished.

Don't get me wrong; I believe in victory. I love the idea of success. I encourage my clients to set goals and visualize achieving them, and then I spend a lot of time and effort inspiring and supporting them on their way to success. *I believe in winning.*

But here's the problem:

The opposite of winning is *losing*—or at least, that's the conventional wisdom.

Winning and losing are more than numbers on a scoreboard or a bathroom scale. They trigger deep biological responses within our brains that make us either happy or sad. Understanding this biology is key to attaining long-term health and happiness.

First, to survive, all animals must adapt their behavior in response to their experiences. Humans are no different. We call this *learning*.

To do this, we need the computational capacity (or brain power) to process the results of our behavior and actions. If you do something that is good for you, your brain measures the benefit, records it, and then integrates the new data and knowledge into your future decisions. [31]

Let's imagine that you decide to have a good night's sleep. That's a healthy thing to do. Your brain records the positive consequences (or *reward*) of the good night's sleep, stores this in your memory, and then serves it up again the next time you debate whether to go to bed early.

Similarly, our brain records, stores, and retrieves bad experiences (or *punishment*) to help inform future decisions. When you place your hand on a hot stove and get burned, your brain logs this event, stores it, and retrieves it next time you're in the proximity of a hot stove.

The simplest form of these complex thought patterns was described in the 19th century by Edward (Ted) Thorndike, a psychologist and researcher from Columbia University, in his "law of effect." [32] You will recognize it as the stimulus-response model used by many subsequent scientists, including the famous Pavlov and his dogs. [33] This law states that each of us has the ability to learn an appropriate response to a specific stimulus. If the outcome is positive, the association between stimulus and response is strengthened; if the outcome is negative, the connection is weakened.

There are far more complex pathways that our powerful brains can process, but it's enough for our purposes to understand this simple stimulus-response framework. And I'm sure that you're beginning to appreciate that the currency of such learning is reward and punishment.

For survival, many choices need to be made instantaneously. Quick action requires an instantaneous evaluation of the potential impact of each possible future action based on both *expected rewards* and *expected punishments*. For less urgent decisions, we get more time to weigh the likely balance of reward and punishment. But the principal is the same: All of our important decisions are forward-looking. Every time we make a decision, we are anticipating either reward or punishment.

The circuitry of reward and the circuitry of punishment, although intimately related, are housed in different parts of the brain. As they drive a critical survival skill, they both reside deep within our primitive, instinctual brains and are among the earliest centers in our brain to have evolved. Both centers are common to all vertebrates[34] (animals with a backbone) and serve as functional links[35] in the brain between the incoming sensory pathways and the outgoing behavioral pathways. Together, the two centers perform mirrored roles[36] in the symmetric reward-punishment system. Favorable stimuli (and the expectation of reward) result in the release of "happy hormones." Unfavorable stimuli (and the expectation of punishment) inhibit the release of "happy hormones."

This element of *expectation*[37] is critical to our understanding of happiness. The reason is simple, if not intuitive. When we expect reward[38] but it doesn't happen, the brain senses this as punishment. Similarly, if we expect punishment and it doesn't happen, the brain registers this as reward. And all this happens at the deep, chemical level.[39]

Whereas both reward and punishment are effective in changing future behavior and habit, I've always been drawn to the superior value of affirmation. In my opinion, affirmation and positive feedback are far more powerful drivers of sustainable behavior change.

I have yet to meet an individual who doesn't respond to affirmation. Even the most hardened and cynical leaders respond to positive feedback.

Imagine the beauty of a world in which each and every one of us was striving to exert an influence only through positivity and affirmation.

That's a world I want to live in.

I'm convinced that this theory has its roots in the fact that the currency of learning is dopamine, the happiness hormone.[40] By dialing this up or down, we learn to modulate future behavior. Mother Nature built a system that fundamentally works via the presence (or absence) of internal chemical affirmation.

To appreciate this, let's go through an exercise that will be familiar to most (if not all) readers. About midday on December 31, each of us starts to consider with a mix of nostalgia and excitement the change that will happen at midnight. Actually, nothing happens in the grand scheme. But we use this nominal turning point to muster energy and resolve for new beginnings. As the afternoon proceeds, we first build, then refine and rank our list of New Year's resolutions. Then, when we finally open our eyes on the morning of January 1, we set out (once again) to exercise, lose weight, be nice, make money…or whatever your favorite resolution might be.

Having read about the biology of reward, you know that, deep in your brain, your reward circuitry has started to expect success. In your cognitive mind's eye, you hold the image of Mr. or Ms. Universe. This is the new person with slim waist and sleek, well-toned limbs that you're going to become. Your reward circuitry is primed for the arrival of this superhero. It stockpiles dopamine so that, when you achieve this goal—when you *win*—it will explode with a powerful surge of chemical happiness reaching the furthest recesses of your affirmation-seeking self!

And what happens in most cases? Well, I don't really need to describe this for you. We're all intimately familiar with the letdown on January 17 when, finally, you acknowledge that you haven't magically morphed into a model of physical perfection. And then Mother Nature unleashes all the venom and anger pent up in your punishment circuitry. Your dopamine gets locked away, and your life enters that horrible cold, dark, lonely corridor.

Sound familiar?

So, what went wrong?

To understand the positive power of expectation, let's look somewhere else. For this example, and because I'm in love with Apple design, we'll choose the Apple laboratories as the setting for this metaphoric story.

What might have happened when Steve Jobs got the first prototype of the cellular phone in his hands? Imagine it weighed about four pounds and needed a small trolley to carry it. Did he throw it to the ground saying, "That's it…we *failed*… there will be no more mobile phones!"?

Well, in all honesty, he may have thrown it to the ground, but I believe that when the engineers regrouped in their lab, they didn't descend into a war of insults and blame. They celebrated.

They knew that they had triumphed in producing the first prototype of something amazing. They knew that they had learned something from the exercise and the feedback. They knew that they would iterate, break down, rebuild, learn, and repeat. After all, they called it the mobile phone 1.0 simply because they knew that 2.0 was not far behind, and it was this iterative journey, this run of small victories that would take them to the ultimate celebration.

What can we learn from the success of Apple's iPhones?

It's simple, and it's about expectations. The ultimate goal of Jobs and his engineers was a sleek, beautiful little handheld device that would connect people across the globe without wires. They never abandoned this vision. But they realized that it would take many steps, many errors (even failures), and many design enhancements before they could deliver the big prize.

If they had seen this as a one-and-done, a win-or-lose, then when the first clunky prototype thudded onto the lab bench, their brains would have yelled in unison that they had failed, and physiological punishment would have followed. Their dopamine would have been shut down and locked away. They would have been miserable, and their creativity would have dried up.

Instead, their reward centers viewed each step as a win, their dopamine reservoirs bursting open with each new version, flooding their brains with joy and leaving them inspired and ready for the next leg of their journey toward success.

So you see, the opposite of winning is not losing, but learning! Don't view life through a win-lose lens. Embrace failure as a vital step on the way to success. This way, you will keep Mother Nature and your powerful brain working with you rather than against you, and you will master the *win-followed-by-win-followed-by-win-until-victory* mindset!

STAYING YOUNG

As I walked along the beach at the end of another beautiful summer in Southern California, I noticed the demographic shift in the tourists who were enjoying the last warm hours of the day's sunshine. Families with older children had returned home to start the new school year, replaced by younger families who were not yet bound by the same calendar.

Everywhere I looked, I saw little bodies running, digging, splashing, and laughing.

A young grandmother ran past me. She was doing her best to keep up with her grandchild, who was enthusiastically charging toward the water's edge.

The little girl's blonde hair flashed behind her—a dancing testimony to unrestrained bliss and youthful zeal. Her pretty face was decorated with a vibrant smile and dancing eyes.

The doting grandparent was grinning as she rushed past me—her life overflowing with ecstasy as the infectious rapture of her tiny prodigy enlivened her own pleasure. She flashed a smile at me and shared these tantalizing words:

"I wish I was four years old again!"

At first, I heard the message with polite amusement. Yes, of course, we all do, I thought.

As I continued my walk, her words sank in, striking deep resonance within me. I turned to look at the crowded beach, and with profound sincerity I said out loud, "Yes, of course—we all do!"

You see, I have realized through both my personal and professional lives that every one of us is involved, throughout our mortal existence, in the earnest pursuit of joy as our highest aspiration. Every client I see today, whether a Fortune 100 CEO looking to be better next year, an Olympic athlete training for a gold medal, or a hard-working parent who comes to me to find courage and direction, is looking for the same thing: happiness.

And there it was, right in front of me. And the grandmother knew it!

Over the past decade, I have come to realize that we are born perfect. Mother Nature designed us to be healthy and happy. I see the evidence as a scientist, as an executive coach, and as a student of life. I see clearly how the modern lifestyle—characterized by sedentary living, overeating, sleep deprivation, and social isolation—is increasingly depriving us of these two birthrights.

More importantly, I see that, when we honor our natural design, we are rewarded with these same two elusive prizes: health and happiness.

We would all do well to not only wish to be four years old again but to study the life of a four-year-old, emulating their instinctive practices…especially on the beach!

To start with, they move. Lots! They seem to respond to a natural drive to keep busy. As their bare feet hit the sand, their legs erupt into wild action. And it's not only their legs. It never ceases to amaze me how children like to dig in the sand. When I walk on the beach, I frequently have to step around a whirl of little arms that are wildly clawing sand out of a hole that is growing in size with each frenzied scoop.

And when did you last try to get a four-year-old to eat? They seem to understand that food is for nourishment and not pleasure. They eat when they're hungry and refuse when they're not, responding to the ache in their belly and not some imaginary ache in their mind.

And have you ever watched a bunch of preschoolers at a birthday party? They are instantly friends with the little ones on either side of them—whether they have met before or not—simply because they are near each other. Community is instinctive for them. Collaboration in fun is their natural disposition.

And, at the end of the day, they collapse with the birds and the setting sun into a deep sleep, to restore body, mind, and spirit. Their carefree rest allows Mother Nature's invisible little helpers to groom connections and remove clutter from growing brains, while repairing and strengthening the organs and limbs that sustain their vital existence.[41]

But that's not all. In fact, this is only half of it. The real magic is taking place deep within their untainted psyches.

At our psychic roots, we are all children. You will often hear people speak fondly of "the child within."[42] That is the simple, trusting, creative, and courageous soul we were born with.

But then life happens. The well-intentioned admonishments and warnings of caring parents and the inevitable traumatic events associated with the human condition systematically induce protective layers that steadily separate us from childhood and childishness. With these steps, we begin the inevitable journey away from innate joy.

Today, I work with adults to understand the myriad of sub-personalities that spawn within them in response to traumas big and small. Distress always induces a protective response. And each time, we bury that innocent, hopeful self a little more.[43]

This may sound like a thoroughly depressing worldview to hold. And if it stopped there, it would be.

But I have learned through my personal life, by studying the world's most composed leaders, and through the amazing transformations of my clients that this is not the path we are condemned to.

There is a better way, and we have a choice.

First, despite the societal pressures that conspire to keep us inactive, overfed, unrested, and isolated, we can choose to pursue daily habits and practices that restore our natural design. The inescapable reward is physical and emotional health.

Second, there are proven techniques for understanding and nurturing our inner psyches. Each one of us can learn to appreciate the complicated mosaic of our inner landscape. Without getting trapped in gloomy or narcissistic introspection, each of us has the capacity to achieve self-mastery, a state wherein we combine the wisdom of the adult with the hopefulness of the child.

If you have never tasted this, the most powerful and rewarding phase of your life remains ahead of you. Once you have experienced it, you will never look back. Your life will become a magnificent journey, as you strive for deeper insight and consciousness while enjoying the fruits of your mortal birthright.

Yes, indeed…there is great value to be found in chasing four-year-olds.

THE CLOWN'S SECRET
TO HAPPINESS

Every circus has a clown. Their role is uplifting. They bring relief and humor, breaking the tension between sword-swallowing, fire-breathing, lion-taming, and high-wire balancing. They interact intimately with the audience, frequently stepping out of the ring to get closer to the wide-eyed children in the front rows.

Clowns laugh out loud. They laugh at their clowning colleagues, the audience, and the cranky ringmaster—but mostly they laugh at themselves. They throw back their heads in loud guffaws before crumpling to the floor, slapping their thighs, as mirth overwhelms them. Even their made-up faces display hilarity, with their plump red noses hinting at their perpetually jolly disposition and their mouths painted in an enduring fleshy grin.

But there is one little feature of the classical clown's face that few notice. He or she always has a little teardrop painted under one or both eyes. According to legend, clowns introduced the tear to remind us that they are real people. Despite their ever-present humor, they also have other feelings. In fact, their wild laughter in performance often hides a melancholy soul, predisposed to sadness and depression. When the flashing lights and loud music subside, the clowns return to their dressing rooms to wipe off their makeup, and with this act they remove the overt signs of their theatrical happiness.

I admit that, as a young boy, I was a little troubled by the clowns. I found their over-the-top hilarity unsettling. As I grew up, though, I developed huge respect for these jokers. Today, I admire their enormous courage and valiant efforts to make our world a better place, to spread the joy that they are so often missing themselves.

We can learn several life lessons from studying these familiar circus characters.

First, our faces are powerful communication tools. We each have 43 muscles in our face, giving us an astounding 8.8 trillion unique facial gestures.[44] We are healthy and happy when we use these, and when we pay close attention to the facial expressions of others. Don't hide behind the phone, email, or text messages. Get out and "into the faces" of family, friends, and colleagues. If you must communicate in writing, use emojis to share your feelings.

Second, humor is both healthy and infectious. A host of good scientific research has proven the tangible health benefits of smiling and laughing.[45] Make sure that you laugh out loud, on occasion falling around like our painted circus friends—even if you do it while nobody is watching. Just as the clown uses humor to break the tension between heavy acts, you can use it to relieve the stresses of a modern life.

Finally, and most importantly, there are times when you must force a smile. Especially when you are at your lowest, the simple physical act of smiling or laughing lifts your mood at a chemical level.[46] Clowns across the ages have known that there are times to fake it until you make it—follow their lead and smile until you mean it.

The clown's contrasting tear and smile capture clues about our real nature—how we all walk a tightrope between joy and suffering, happiness and sadness. I hope that the clown's face will inspire you to study and emulate their strategy. Each of us can systematically build joy in our lives and the lives of those around us by acting positively—and even forcing a happy face, if necessary.

BOOSTING CONFIDENCE

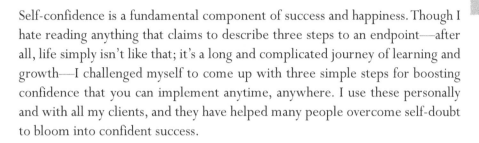

Self-confidence is a fundamental component of success and happiness. Though I hate reading anything that claims to describe three steps to an endpoint—after all, life simply isn't like that; it's a long and complicated journey of learning and growth—I challenged myself to come up with three simple steps for boosting confidence that you can implement anytime, anywhere. I use these personally and with all my clients, and they have helped many people overcome self-doubt to bloom into confident success.

1. Identify Your Top Three Strengths

Too often, a loss of confidence leaves us feeling that we're losers. But we aren't. Even Olympians have temporary slumps in confidence. But when they remember the strengths that got them to the top of their game, they have a good chance of regaining their mojo.

To remember your own strengths, I recommend a simple, fun exercise. Set aside a few minutes each morning and evening for a full week to jot down three things about yourself that you are most proud of. It might be your intelligence, or your sense of humor, or your determination or creativity, or something else that is uniquely and powerfully you. At the end of the week, look over the output of this exercise and see which three strengths appeared on your daily entries most often. These are the three things somebody who knows you well would probably identify as your strengths, and you can be proud of each one.

This focused self-insight is important because awareness of your specific strengths boosts your overall sense of self-value.

2. Be Thankful for Your Strengths

Especially when you're being hard on yourself, or feeling down, get into the habit of "gratitude musings." Think deeply about your top three strengths and appreciate the profound consequences of each. If you selected your sense of humor, for example, think about how it brings joy and light to the lives of your friends and family. Think about how their laughs and smiles elevate your own mood.

I advise my clients to take long walks while they practice their "gratitude musings." As you walk, go through your strengths one by one. Hold each one in your mind. First, start with just the word. Say it over and over again. Next, define what it means to you. Then describe what it does for you, the many magnificent moments it has earned you. Finally, describe what your gift does for other people, the many wonderful ways you have touched the lives of others with this gift.

When you truly appreciate the value of each of your strengths, your steps will lighten and the clouds will lift.

Remember, gratitude is a powerful force for boosting self-confidence!

3. Flood Your Brain with Positivity

All three parts of our brain have a voice, and our attitude at any particular moment is dictated by which voice is loudest.

If you're low in self-confidence, it is because your voice of fear is dominant.

To dilute that voice of fear, flood your mind with positive thoughts and emotions. This is a powerful way to boost your confidence. Use mantras, motivating words, and positive images to remember your many victories. All of these infuse positivity into your cognitive brain.

And positive thoughts drive confidence!

A TRUE LESSON
IN GENIUS

There is an apocryphal story about the great American inventor Thomas Edison.[47]

He returned home from school one day with a letter from his teacher. She had given him very strict instructions: He was not to open the letter, and he was not to share it with anybody other than his mother.

Little Thomas was a good, hardworking boy, so he carried the letter home and carefully delivered it to his mother.

A little surprised and fearing the worst, she took the letter into her bedroom, where she opened and read it. She emerged several minutes later. With tears in her eyes, she read the letter out loud to Thomas.

She told him how his teacher thought that he was a genius—that he was too intelligent to be educated at his current school and she recommended that Mrs. Edison keep the young boy at home, to teach him herself.

Thomas Edison went on to become one of the world's great inventors.[48] *He famously captured the power of electricity in the world's first light bulb. He built the original phonogram that later became the earliest gramophone. He produced the world's first motion pictures. With over a thousand patents to his name, few people would argue with the claim that he was a true genius.*

Now, the story continues that Thomas returned to his childhood home after his mother's death. He spent an afternoon sifting through her papers, tidying up her estate.

He came across a neatly folded envelope that he recognized to be the letter he brought home from school that day. Filled with pride and happy memories, he opened the letter. For the first time, with his own eyes, he read the two short sentences his teacher had written to his mother:

> *"Thomas is addled. He can no longer attend this school."*
>
> *The old Thomas closed his eyes for a long time. When he opened them, he took a clean sheet of paper from his mother's desk and wrote his own simple conclusion:*
>
> *"Thomas Edison was an addled child who, by the heroic actions of his mother, became the genius of the 19th century."*

Like all apocryphal stories, this one caught the public's attention because it just could have been true. More importantly, for me, it clearly illustrates the immense power of belief.

Regardless of the authenticity of this story, I hope you take it to heart. Whether you're a parent of young children, a 43-year-old reinventing yourself, or a millennial with much of your adult life still ahead of you, the message is crystal clear: You are a genius…so be it!

LESSONS IN HAPPINESS FROM A FURRY FRIEND

I was walking up the steep path that led away from the beach. Deep in thought, I hardly noticed the woman walking toward me. As she got closer, I suddenly noticed the face of her dog.

He was a short-haired English Labrador—the ones with the big broad head and deep brown eyes. He was a sturdy fellow, in his prime. He bustled along next to his owner, his tail wagging behind him and his ears slightly cocked in excitement. He held his head close to her knee as they moved briskly down the hill in my direction.

And then it struck me.

His mouth was wrinkled into a smile that radiated pure, unrestrained happiness. Yes, the dog was smiling. And if you've seen a Lab like this, you'll know that it was a real, unmistakable smile.

And this got me thinking…

For some reason, most of the Labradors I know are inclined to smile. It may be something unique to the breed, which has a highly affable reputation.[49] It may also have to do with the nature of the species, known as "man's best friend."

So, I started to think about their neurobiology, and the gift they have that may be the reason for this joyful disposition. This beautiful Lab was overflowing with social instincts from the emotional brain and displayed them readily in his facial expression.

My next realization was even more powerful. I was struck by how different this dog's life was than the life of an average human being. Few of us run around grinning from ear to ear all day.

Why?

Too often, we become our own best enemies. And at those times, our cognitive brains wipe away our smiles.

We are the ones who impose boundaries, seed doubts and fears, and sabotage our own plans. Our powers of thought and imagination are powerful assets when deployed with positivity, but we are highly vulnerable to self-doubt.

So, why are dogs so happy? Because they have enough advanced brain to get away from the cold life of a lizard but not enough to get trapped in *self-destructive ideation*.

What a gift.

So, what's my take-home for all of us?

First, remember to smile. It's a powerful tool that drives your own health and happiness and spreads positivity into the lives of others.

Second, take a good look at your life. Are you feeling happy right now? Are you achieving success in the big and important things: family, health, career?

If your answer to any of these is "no," then take your courage in both hands, take a good, long look inside your powerful mind, and ask yourself a very important question: "Is there something that I have created within my powerful cognitive brain that is keeping me from health, happiness, and prosperity?"

When we remove the fear and doubt that originate in our primitive brain and are amplified by our cognitive brain, we have the best chance of being happy.

I hope this happy dog inspires you to take action today!

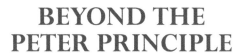

BEYOND THE PETER PRINCIPLE

Too often we run up against false boundaries in our personal and professional lives, limiting our performance and keeping us from our full executive potential. I am convinced that the infamous Peter Principle has played a role in these destructive circumstances.

On my way up the professional ladder, I was periodically troubled by the prospect of waking up one day in a senior role that was one step beyond my natural talents. I reflected on how miserable it would be to be trapped by my own success, thrust into a role laden with expectations I couldn't hope to meet.

Laurence Peter and Raymond Hull famously ushered the "Peter Principle" into the corporate lexicon in 1969 when they released their book of the same name.[50]

Formally stated, the Peter Principle proclaims that people in a hierarchy tend to rise to the level of their own incompetence.

It is not clear if Peter and Hull's book was intended for entertainment or as a serious guide for corporate architects and ambitious executives. It may very well have been written as a satire rather than a business manual.

Either way, the Peter Principle has tiptoed through the boardrooms of organizational life for over 50 years, preying on unsuspecting corporate executives and employees alike.[51]

It is easy to understand the origins of the principle: a combination of widespread managerial incompetence, the knowledge that junior-level talent doesn't always translate into executive performance, and the endemic fear of being exposed as an imposter. But what is less clear is its value.

At best, it provides a humorous view of organizational disaster and perhaps helps us explain some of the frustration we feel when we're exposed to an incompetent manager. At worst, it has fertilized a rampant self-doubt epidemic and has precipitated untold human suffering through its evil cousin, the imposter syndrome.

Interestingly, through my personal life and my time as a professional coach, I have learned that there is a phenomenon far more terrifying than the Peter Principle.

It is *fear* of the Peter Principle.

I have absolutely no doubt that the prevalence of grievous career damage is more often the result of deep apprehension about the limits of our own competence than the result of any real limits that exist.

How do I know this?

I work with courageous men and women who seek my guidance in their quest for peak performance. We work together to identify their limiting beliefs and then leap beyond them using a systematic, science-based coaching methodology.

The process reignites their confidence and passion and liberates them from their own perceived performance limits in dramatic fashion. They surge forward into a life fully supported by their own abundant competence.

As a result, I am ready to declare the end of the Peter Principle. The increasing depths of personal insight in the liberated modern corporate worker have made the principle redundant—a beautiful irony, in that it has itself fallen victim to its own prophesy. Said otherwise, it has risen to the level of its own incompetence.

It is now time for each of us to turn inward to address the roadblocks we put on our own paths and to emerge as victors, striding forward beyond the Peter Principle in renewed vitality and confidence.

BE WHO
YOU WANT TO BE

We need to get out of our own way. Only *we* stand between our current reality and our future desires. Think about it…

Do you want to be happy? I bet you do. I want to be happy, and every one of my clients does, too.

> *Who is stopping you?*
>
> *The truth is, nobody is stopping you.*
>
> *If you want to be happy, be happy.*
>
> *If you want to laugh, then laugh.*
>
> *If you want to be adventurous, be adventurous.*
>
> *If you want to be creative, be creative.*
>
> *If you want to be calm, be calm.*
>
> *Who is stopping you?*

Throughout our lives, we acquire reasons to act in ways that oppose our deep desires. We gain something by being sad, angry, cautious, chaotic, frenzied, or needy.

For example, many of my CEO clients are addicted to their work. Despite their profound desire for peace and calm, their lives seem to explode each day into feverish activity. They feel such activity has brought them success, but many of them also bemoan children who have grown up, or even grown away, as they themselves fought their way to professional victory.

Or, consider the sad little boy who used his melancholy to gain the attention he so desperately needed when he was growing up. Perhaps he was the child of parents addicted to busyness. Either way, sadness served his purposes well. But it has now lasted into adulthood, and he can't escape its devastating grasp on his life.

Being sad, angry, cautious, chaotic, frenzied, and needy has side effects. They might get us to our short-term goals, but those states lack the enduring power to illuminate our journey to more meaningful destinations.

Worse still, they entrap us. We become stuck in rigid mindsets that keep us from achieving the happiness we so desperately desire.

I work closely with individual clients to understand the origins and motives of the stubbornly enduring mindsets that keep them from their goals. We learn to unravel hard-wired behavior patterns that once secured their short-term survival. These courageous women and men liberate themselves from the bondage of deeply entrenched survival mindsets to find the lasting clarity and joy they deserve.

But I sometimes think we make things too complicated.

If you want to be happy…then just be happy!

Nobody is stopping you but you.

MINDSETS
TO THRIVE

TAMING FEAR TO SUCCEED

Do you daydream? You know, those beautiful, hazy moments when you allow your imagination to run free? What do you picture?

Floating on a crystal-clear, sparkling blue ocean in brilliant sunshine? Cruising in a shiny red sports car? The perfect home, with the perfect family, including the clean-up-after-itself, non-shedding dog? Smiling children—healthy and happy?

And then do you bump back down into your real life only to find that you're stuck in traffic, waiting for a train, staring out of your cubicle, or sitting at your laptop while the rest of the family is fast asleep?

What would you give to switch back into that dream world—this time for real?

In truth, you can always get a lot closer to that dream than you think you can… or, more precisely, *if* you think you can! But you're going to have to change a few things.

Yes, that's right—you're going to have to change. You can't get *there* from *here*.

Change can be hard, especially big change. But why is it that change is so difficult, even painful, for most of us?

Well, for a start, you may not have understood that you're fighting against a natural enemy within yourself. It's called *fear*. It takes immense courage to release your grasp on the security of the old, trusting that the new is waiting to catch you on the other side.

Sadly, in life, many people never let go of the security of the old. Regardless of their draw to the new, or even the misery they are going through stuck in the old, their fear of the release is too strong. For many, it's easier to maintain the status quo.

Fear is a powerful force, originating deep within your primitive brain, and it is a powerful opponent of change, even when that change is for the better.

Your primitive brain surfaces fear in several recognizable guises. Once you understand and acknowledge their origin, you should be able to actively engage your cognitive and emotional brains to overcome fear and doubt, allowing you to embrace change.

Here are several common presentations of fear:

The fear of pain or discomfort (including effort). This fear is frighteningly common because it is closest to the original purpose of the reptilian brain: to protect us against physical danger. Your primitive brain quickly alerts you to the pain of having to move to a new city if you get the promotion or the new job, or the chances of getting your heart broken as you begin a new relationship. It works to preserve the safe, familiar status quo. But are you really going to run out of physical energy while you launch the new business or start that new non-profit to help others?

The fear of failure. More complex to understand, this fear still boils down to a simple principle: Your reptilian brain wants to protect you from public humiliation—or worse, humiliation in front of *yourself.* You're not really afraid of failure; you're afraid of its consequences. But the truth is that, although such fear is somewhat logical, you tend to exaggerate both the likelihood and the negative consequences of failure. Would you really be the only person to ever miss out on the leading role in that sold-out-forever Broadway musical?

The fear of effort. Few valuable things are attained without effort. It's unlikely that you are genuinely lazy and truly afraid of hard work itself. Instead, I believe that your primitive brain surfaces this fear to protect you from deeper concerns. If you're telling yourself it's too hard to achieve your dreams, dig a little deeper. You will probably find one of the other fears lurking there, disguising itself as the fear of effort. Because has a little hard work ever hurt you?

The fear of criticism. None of us like being criticized, and if you suspect that this will be the reward for your efforts, you may be afraid to try something new. Again, your reptilian brain wants to protect you against harsh words that hurt—and, by the way, they really do hurt. But how many people do you know who have been thrown out of society for running in the mayoral election?

The fear of the unknown. Instinctively, we are cautious of the unknown. Yes, it's true that there will be many new things you will have to encounter and master on the way to the life of your dreams…and most of them you cannot anticipate. But look back over your life. How many unexpected obstacles have you already faced and overcome?

The fear of success. This is the hardest to understand, yet alarmingly common, and it can be profoundly debilitating. There are two obvious reasons we fear success: Firstly, success will change us, especially if we achieve our biggest dreams. Picture the dream that you have placed outside of your own reach. Imagine if you had already achieved it. Life would be different, right? But why should this frighten you? It's true: If you move to a tropical paradise, you really will have to leave this dirty old home that you've sweated and invested in, where your children were born and raised. But, hey…you seem to have forgotten how brilliantly the sunshine shimmered off those blue waves as you floated effortlessly on your dreamy ocean!

I don't mean in any way to belittle the fears that rip you harshly out of your daydreams. I know that those fears are real, painful, and hard to overcome. But I am trying to illustrate a few simple points:

First, it's helpful to acknowledge the source of your fear. After all, it's an entirely natural and healthy part of who we are. I even recommend that you thank your reptilian brain. Thank it for wanting to keep you safe!

But then you must move on. Do not allow the negative voice to keep the upper hand.

Move quickly to questioning its rationale. What is the real likelihood of your failing? Are the consequences really as dire as you imagine them to be? Will it really hurt you if somebody ridicules you for trying?

If the voice of fear is still winning over solid reasoning, then it's time to kick your campaign into a higher gear. It's time to bring some mental muscle into the game. It's time to rebuke that unreasonable, limiting fear. Invoke the power of your cognitive brain. Say bold words, hold encouraging thoughts, and paint pictures of success in your mind. The power of positive thought and belief is immense! Study it. Practice it. Use it.

It's important that you remember through all of this that you are not rebuking or challenging yourself. You're not the bad guy. It's just that your reptilian brain is doing too good a job of protecting you. You're strong enough to handle a little risk and a little pain. You're not weak or timid. You've just been listening too attentively to that primitive, protective voice.

Finally, if that negative voice is still keeping you from your dreams, you need to distract it. Find things to be busy with, so you're no longer controlled by fear and doubt. And the best way to do this is to get on building the road to your dreams.

You'll look back after a day of hard work, surprised to realize how little you heard the negative voice and how much progress you made toward your dream.

Every one of my clients comes to me with two common aspirations: First, they want to be happy. Second, they want change...and often, this is the big reason they've sought me out. Change isn't easy. Whether they're in a desperate situation—fighting a messy divorce, trying to find their purpose, or simply overwhelmed by the frenzy of life—or they've come to me to be the best person they can be, our journey together is about change.

Change is always possible. Understand it, embrace it, be brave about it—and the reward is yours for the taking!

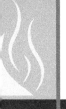

THREE LIBERATING REASONS TO FACE YOUR FEARS

Like many children, I once feared the dark. Even at my young age, though, I realized that my fear was both disproportional and dysfunctional. Fear robbed me of many safe, fun experiences.

One day, I decided to address this limit head on.

I forced myself out into my parents' back garden on the darkest nights. I explored the scariest recesses behind the giant hydrangea bushes. I was determined to prove to myself that the scary things I feared did not exist.

Night after night, I ignored my heart pounding in my chest, clenched my fists to stop my hands from shaking, and strode out into the most menacing corners of our property. No flashlight. No weapon. Not even a stick. I simply armed myself with the knowledge that, despite the haunting presence of vivid images of grotesque danger, these fears existed in my mind, and not in my home.

It worked.

Of course, I still walk down dark alleys in big cities with appropriate caution, but I am no longer a prisoner in my own bedroom when the sun sets.

I am 100% certain that this story will resonate with every reader. Perhaps you were similarly afraid of the dark. Maybe you conquered your fear…or maybe not? Perhaps some other monster has dominated your life, with either personal or professional consequences. You might be afraid of flying, or public speaking, or sharks and snakes, or spiders, or cyber terrorism, or rejection.

Each of us is kept from being our best by our fears.

Today, as a scientist focused on performance and the huge role that health and happiness play in our overall success, I understand the neuroscience of fear. I have come a long way since I was that little boy walking outside in the dark.

More than ever, my advice to you is to face your fears head on. Here is why:

1. Most of your fears are not real.

When I imagined the horrendous atrocities that would befall me in my childhood garden, it was my primitive brain trying to protect me.

The problem is that, if we do not oppose the fearful messages of our primitive brain, the other parts of our brain exaggerate these dangers in both magnitude and perceived consequence. So, an event with a tiny likelihood becomes a strong possibility in our minds, and the consequence of danger becomes unreasonably magnified.

Challenging your fears keeps your brain aware of what is a real threat and what is not, leaving you unfettered by anxiety over imagined dangers.

2. Confronting your fear is a profound source of self-insight.

The cognitive brain not only provides us with the means to counteract our fears, but it also empowers us with insight. Unfortunately, most of us don't give it a chance to do those things. A natural consequence of fear is avoidance. Nobody enjoys the real physical and emotional pain associated with fear. So, we avoid them.

On the other hand, when we seek out our fears, corner them, and focus our massive cognitive powers on their bare threads, we see them for what they really are.

Self-insight is the second step to liberation.

3. Conquering your fear is a powerful growth driver.

We find very clever ways to avoid confronting our fears.

If you're afraid of public speaking, for example, you are likely to contrive reasons why your shyness is not really that limiting: "I can build a successful career without speaking...most people just get up there and blabber anyway...mostly, we communicate through email...some of the most famous authors are shy, reclusive geniuses."

Yes, there are many roles in life that do not require public speaking to be successful. But, there are millions of people around the world whose lives would be transformed if they could expand beyond their unreasonably limiting fears.

I've worked with enough clients, patients, and colleagues to know that every human being has unrealized potential and that the single biggest barrier to unleashing this potential is fear.

I invite you to learn more about fear, limiting thoughts, and, most importantly, the liberating power of belief. I hope that you will do this with renewed determination and confidence.

Remember: At the end of the day, most fears are only a little, primitive voice inside your head.

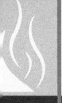

REFLEX NEGATIVITY:
A SLIPPERY SLOPE

The other day, I was rummaging in the refrigerator when an egg fell out and shattered on the floor at my feet. To the sound of loud self-abuse, I grabbed a roll of paper towels and began to clean up the mess. Crawling around on the floor, I mentally berated myself: "You're stupid! How could you have been so careless? What kind of idiot lets things fall out of the fridge? Like you didn't have enough to deal with today already?"

What happens immediately after you drop something? What are the first words that come out of your mouth? Do they help you or hurt you?

Reflexes are immediate responses that are so quick they bypass the processing centers in your brain.[52] As a physician, I would test my patients' peripheral nerve reflexes often—you've probably experienced that knee-jerk test yourself, when your physician taps your kneecap with a little rubber hammer.

These tests are useful in showing the function of the brain and other elements of your nervous system, precisely because you can't control them. Your cognitive override (overthinking brain) is sidelined for a moment, and we get to see the raw state of your underlying neurological health.

Perhaps examining our emotional reflexes would be helpful, too.

If you're anything like me, the first word that comes out of your mouth after you drop something is too profane to print here. But that's not the word I'm really interested in…it's the words that follow the expletive that shed light on your fundamental wiring.

Again, if you're anything like me, the next words tend to be highly personal and highly critical—something like, "I'm so stupid" or "I'm such a clumsy idiot!"

Here is what I learn from this response:

First, it signals a default state of mind that is negative, even self-critical.

Second, and more worrying by far, is that this deep reflex is self-perpetuating. You see, we actually believe what we're telling ourselves. The intensely negative reflex statement, which may seem more like a release of pressure than an impactful message, goes back into our brains at both the cognitive and the emotional levels and breeds more negativity and self-criticism. We get trapped in an ever-intensifying and destructive feedback loop.

This danger is exacerbated by three characteristics of the reflex statement. First, it's very *personal*. There is no doubt that we single ourselves out as the miserable, defective culprit. Second, the statement is *pervasive*. It implies that we are stupid or clumsy across every domain of our lives. Third, the accusation is *permanent*. We don't limit the insult to the current moment in time. We simply say "I'm stupid," which means that that we're *always* stupid.

Of course, we don't really mean all those bad things about ourselves. But the words are absorbed that way by our very receptive brains whether we like it or not. That reflex statement is a damning message of personal, pervasive, and permanent fault.

So how do we escape this reflex negativity and its resultant longer-term pessimism? The good news is that this is possible. Pioneers of optimism and positive psychology, like Martin Seligman of the University of Pennsylvania, have demonstrated the power of positive interventions.[53]

Seligman proposes three ways of managing negative responses to bad events[54]:

1. **Disputation.** Argue with yourself. In my example, I clearly don't believe that I'm stupid, so I must strike that word and replace it with something more accurate and less damning. Find examples that refute what you've said in your self-abusive statement. You have to point out that the statement is simply not true.

2. **Distraction.** This is particularly helpful over the longer term. If you are brooding over a bad work situation or personal life crisis, you may find yourself repeatedly saying things like, "I'm useless," or "Nobody likes me." These are deeply rooted, emotionally loaded explanations, which are also personal, pervasive, and permanent. If your disputation is not working, then call a time-out. Distract yourself with something else (action is a great distraction). It may be helpful to agree to address the underlying issue later in the week, giving yourself time to arrive at a more balanced perspective and perhaps come up with a couple of good arguments against your current undermining explanation.

3. Distance. I love this one, and it's subtly different than distraction. The best description of this technique is a beautiful question that Seligman uses with his pessimistic clients. He asks them, "What would you say if a disheveled drunk in the street said the same thing to you?" I can picture this dirty, drunk person looking at me through bloodshot eyes, yelling, "You're stupid!" It would take me no more than half a second before I had a long list of arguments disputing that preposterous statement. Or, even better, I would simply ignore it.

I hope that this little snapshot helps you to think about the way you react to adversity and, in particular, the words that you use to explain the seemingly bad events that we all experience every day. It has a real impact on your health and happiness, and you can improve it with practice. Invest some time in scrutinizing your explanations and expletives. Identify when you are being inappropriately and reflexively personal, pervasive, and permanent in your negativity and self-criticism. Challenge yourself, distract yourself, and, if necessary, get dirty and distance yourself.

Which brings me back to your reflex negativity. Next time you drop the glass jar as you take it out of the refrigerator, listen to your words. They will tell you how you're doing on your road to happiness and success.

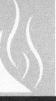

FREE YOURSELF FROM
A DESTRUCTIVE MINDSET

Once upon a time, our daily existence was consumed by a desperate struggle for survival.

Homo sapiens was not yet born. Our ancestors were little more than animals. To be honest, we were biologically indistinguishable from the rest of the animal kingdom. To help us endure the threats of a savage planet, where only the strongest survived, Mother Nature built us a powerful brain. Moving from battle to battle, our primitive brain was fueled by a combination of fear and the primal knowledge that we simply *had* to win.

And it worked!

It worked so well, in fact, that those early ancestors began a 60-million-year journey toward today. Thanks to this polarized win-lose mindset, you are now living comfortably as a modern person in the 21st century.

But something changed.

This profound but subtle change has been noticed by some of the world's most powerful thinkers. Rudyard Kipling, the 19th-century English writer born in India and most famous for *The Jungle Book*, reveals his insight in these two lines from his well-known poem "If—"[55]:

> *If you can meet with Triumph and Disaster*
>
> *and treat those two impostors just the same*
>
> *…then…*
>
> *Yours is the Earth and everything that is in it.*

Surprisingly, in these lines of this poem, he dismisses the very instinct that enabled our ancestors to survive. Almost contemptuously, he labels victory and defeat as "imposters." He identifies them as unwelcome intruders that keep us from achieving our dreams.

As I hear these lines again, I am reminded of so many of my clients.

The 27-year-old millionaire who is desperately unhappy as he heads off in search of the next million. The 54-year-old who has not experienced a day of fulfillment after her retirement as an international endurance athlete 26 years ago. The 43-year-old breadwinner who has been crippled by his belief that his recent pay cut proves he is a failure. The couple in their late thirties who fight incessantly because they believe that, if they do not win each argument, they will lose. All of these examples show how prevalent the win-lose mindset still is.

But, today, the prevailing concepts of Triumph and Disaster are redundant and harmful. We no longer need these deep survival instincts, yet they persist with disastrous consequences.

The two bookends of Triumph and Disaster insert themselves prematurely on the continuum of possibility. When we achieve a victory, there is always something bigger and better we could have achieved. Indeed, when we fail, there is always a greater failure we could contemplate, a greater depth we could reach.

The concepts of Triumph and Disaster grossly limit our potential.

Using your full brain, you will recognize that both Triumph and Defeat are limiting and destructive illusions. If you realize this, you will be in a position to realize your highest potential. You will become *unstoppable*.

For your complete success, focus on the "new" skills we have acquired as a species. Find the stillness of your prefrontal cortex and contemplate all the forces affecting our present moment, including fears, feelings, and thoughts. Then—and not before then—you can rise above the ruthless grip of fear and become master of your own destiny.

What will you do today to ensure you realize your immense potential?

How will you reject the limits induced by fear?

How will you learn to use your greatest gift, your full brain, to become *unstoppable*?

Kipling's poem ends with a massive, irresistible promise: "Yours is the Earth, and everything that is in it." Kipling drops this tantalizing hope at the end of a long list of challenging preconditions. *If* you do this, and that, and the next thing… *then*…you can have anything you want.

I wish you "the Earth, and everything that is in it" as you push past victory and defeat to realize your fullest potential.

A ROCKY PATH
TRIGGERS CHANGE

The foundation of physical health and happiness is movement—and lots of it. It's the first step on the road to abundance. So, when feasible, I hold my meetings with clients walking outside in the sunshine. It was during one of these sessions that Mother Nature gifted me with this illuminating insight.

We were walking high on the cliffs overlooking the Pacific Ocean in Southern California. The path was craggy, with breathtaking views over sparkling seas. My client was walking more slowly than usual. I had slowed down a couple of times, anxious to be responsive to her comfort and needs. About halfway through the walk, she shared with me the reason for her labored gait: Her foot was aching; she felt pain with each step.

She hadn't noticed this pain before, so we sat down while she removed her shoe. She was wearing light, flexible running shoes, the kind with those spongy corrugated soles that open up as you flex them. As we turned the shoe over, the source of her discomfort became immediately apparent. There was a large round hole right under the ball of her foot, where sharp rocks could easily apply direct pressure to her sensitive sole.

But it was the origin of the problem that truly fascinated me.

Several weeks earlier, she had noticed a little stone wedged into the corrugations of her shoe. At first, it was mildly uncomfortable, but she had not bothered to remove it. Instead, she chose to walk on with that slightly irritating clicking noise each time the stone hit the hard surface of the road. In due course, she forgot about it.

After several weeks, the stone had become an entrenched part of her shoe, accompanying her every time she exercised. She didn't even notice the regular click-step, click-step, click-step cadence that likely annoyed her fellow walkers.

The day before our session, her elderly father had noticed the stone in her shoe. Before she set out to get her 10,000 steps, he had suggested that she remove it. She pried it out with a strong stick, leaving a gaping hole where the hard stone had crushed the surrounding material.

As we walked back to the base of the cliffs, I thought how ironic it was that life had served her up a physical analogy to help her navigate a big change.

It so happened that she had been contemplating some major changes in her life. I could see her courage growing each week, but she remained one big step away from taking the plunge. We'd been working to identify and address the fears that were stopping her.

I'm sure that you recognize this pattern. At some point, you become aware of a problem. Let's say you're putting on weight or eating more than you should (or, more often, both). Perhaps you have started to rely on an evening drink or you're yelling at your children in response to escalating stress from all that's going on in the world. You note the problem, and then continue your life without really addressing it. The problem then disappears from your awareness, merging into the background of frenetic activity that characterizes our modern lives.

Until somebody else notices it.

At that stage, you're in trouble, because not only do you feel the disruption, but you realize that the solution is likely to be painful. You have grown accustomed to the stone in your shoe. Removing it will leave a gaping hole. And so, most of the time, many of us will ignore the problem again, hoping that somehow it will magically disappear.

By that time, it is too late for the most obvious solution: to avoid the problem in the first place. In the case of my client, if she had reacted appropriately when she first noticed the problem, she could have removed the stone before her shoe was damaged.

Since that was no longer an option, what she needed was to quickly fill the gap she had created with something healthy. She went home and found a little of that magical foam plumbers use to fill cracks and crevices. It provided temporary relief for the damaged shoe.

This simple fix led her very quickly to understand the solution to her bigger problems.

She gathered the courage required to make the big change in her life that she had been avoiding. She quit her job and volunteered at the local homeless shelter while she looked for her next career opportunity. Rather than sitting around at home with a big hole in her life, leaving her vulnerable to the consequences of boredom and purposelessness, she filled the gap before it became a problem.

Today, several years later, she is a powerful leader of a multimillion-dollar company and guides her team to embrace change early, before gaps appear.

I hope that this simple story helps you think about a change that you need to make. Understand the source of your fear. Identify the hole you will create, and find a way to fill it before it becomes a problem. Then step out, embrace the change, and surge forward on your path to victory.

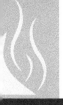

AVOIDING THE
BURNOUT CLIFF

Are you feeling tired, jaded, stale, fatigued, or burned out? These are all common terms used to describe the physical and emotional consequences of overwork.

How can you prevent and, if necessary, recover from this depressing state?

Stress is actually a good force. Without it, we would neither perform nor grow. If you study a normal performance curve, you will notice how increasing your workload, or the stress that drives you to work, actually improves your performance.[56] Then the law of diminishing return kicks in at some point. At that point, additional effort produces only marginal improvement in performance, and stress eventually becomes distress.[57]

Central to this well-described natural phenomenon is the balance of work (or training) and recovery. Athletes know this well. They stress their muscles during training in order to make them stronger, but they must allow them time to recover and build before stressing them again.[58]

This is not only true for our bodies but for our brains and psyche, too. That's why we need sleep. Sleeping or resting too little impairs performance.[59] Each of us must find the highly individualized, optimal ratio of work to rest that drives our sustainable peak performance.

It sounds easy, right? Work harder and harder and then back off to find your high-performance "zone."

Well, it's not. And that's why all too many senior executives, well-known artists and entertainers, and competitive athletes burn out. And it's why so many of us today are feeling increasingly exhausted.

The problem is that the performance curve suddenly and without warning gives way to a massive and precipitous drop.[60] You step over the edge at your peril. One step too many is enough to have you hurtling down toward the base of the cliff. It's a painful ride, and the long way back up is excruciating.

Wisdom comes from knowing how to push yourself as far as possible without actually falling off the edge. I'm sure that you'd like to learn this massive secret, right?

Here's the problem: Our ability to predict the exact location of the edge is sadly lacking. In my personal experience, most elite athletes have fallen off the performance cliff at least once. That's probably also true for anybody who's particularly driven at work.

There *may* be subtle warning signs, but unfortunately, the science is not strong enough for me to claim this unequivocally for all people.

Here is the science about the warning zone[61]: This is the zone where *stress* becomes *distress*, where you begin to experience physical, physiological, emotional, and/or psychological discomfort. Sleep disruption is the most common symptom of distress, expressed as difficulty in falling asleep, increased wakefulness through the night, or reduced quality of sleep. All result in feeling tired on waking.

You can imagine a negative cycle developing rapidly, where distress results in sleep disruption that in turn impairs performance. Competitive people react by increasing their workload to offset the poor performance, precipitating a downward spiral. This is the quick route over the edge of the cliff.

Another physical measure that regularly alerts us to overtraining in athletes is resting heart rate.[62] It is a strong warning signal when this starts to creep up. We also know that cortisol, the body's stress hormone, tends to drop as you burn out. The adrenal system, responsible for your fight and flight reactions, becomes fatigued and under-responsive.

I advise all my clients to systematically monitor their resting heart rate. Over time, this can help us understand their unique physiologic disposition to stress, as a sustained increase in this parameter warrants decisive protective measures.

Perhaps the biggest danger of the warning zone is that a relatively small stress can nudge you over the edge of the cliff. You may be aware that you are in the danger zone but feel confident because you know how close to the edge you are, when an unexpected insult suddenly throws you over the side. The insult may be a minor illness or a seemingly trivial falling out with a friend. I liken this to standing on an actual cliff, when a sudden gust of wind appears to bring the cliff closer toward you—and over you go!

Only a tiny minority of people are able to grab onto a ledge of the cliff on their way down. For the most part, it's a quick, painful descent all the way to the bottom.

After that, the only way back to the top is a long walk back up your original pathway, often requiring a convalescent period before that climb is possible.

The best approach to burnout is prevention.

Listen very carefully to your body. Push through minor resistance, but listen for persistent warnings.

Track your sleep. Track your resting heart rate. Nobody knows your body like you do, and everybody's performance curve is unique (and can change over time). Superhuman ideation is both dangerous and arrogant.

Science is deaf to the protests of heroes as they fall off the cliff. If you hear warning signs, back up a little; reduce your workload; increase your rest and recovery. And then back up one step further. You need to have some extra space between you and the edge to account for the unexpected.

If you do this, you will be able to hold your head high, with a light step and cheery outlook in your zone of maximal performance. You can be your best, for longer. This is how you will secure long-term health and happiness.

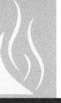

ESCAPE INNER CONFLICT

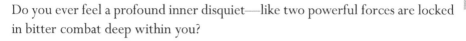

Do you ever feel a profound inner disquiet—like two powerful forces are locked in bitter combat deep within you?

This is the result of a strange quirk in the blueprint of our magnificent human brain. We may even consider it a design flaw, because it causes modern humans a great deal of anguish.

I can't explain *why* we ended up in this predicament, but I can explain *how*. It is the consequence of Mother Nature's iterative design process, otherwise known as evolution.

You see, your reptilian brain works incessantly to keep you safe both physically and emotionally. Since the reptilian brain has primary responsibility for such essential work, it has a very loud voice and is inclined to hijack and direct your full mental capacity.

While your reptilian brain builds structures that ensure your survival by keeping you safe, your cognitive brain simultaneously strives for growth and improvement, giving you a deep-seated biological urge to expand beyond those safe castle walls.

Unfortunately, because of this push-and-pull design, you end up feeling trapped within your own safe prison.

Fortunately, you can take several simple steps to manage this painful conflict that is inherent in our natural design.

Insight: When you understand your natural design, you appreciate the source of the tension. You no longer assume that there is something uniquely and embarrassingly wrong with you.

Control: The knowledge that this is self-imprisonment is itself liberating. It means that you hold the keys to the prison. Your future is in your own hands!

Evolutionary Advantage: Happily, Mother Nature has equipped human beings with a supremely powerful prefrontal cortex. This region of your brain, which fills out the backward-sloping forehead of the great apes, gives you awareness of your awareness, also known as metacognition. When you exploit this gift (through meditation, mindfulness, and other neurological practices), you can experience your thoughts and emotions without being controlled by them.

Personal Mastery: Those who invest time and energy into self-optimization know that it is difficult to fully appreciate your own inner workings. It is always helpful to get an outside-in perspective with the help of a coach trained in neuroscience.

So, if you're troubled by profound inner disquiet—a deep frustration or pain that is difficult to put your finger on—know that it is indeed because there are two powerful forces locked in bitter combat deep within you. Luckily, a little knowledge of our magnificent neurobiology and a few simple, practical steps can help you to escape this persistent, seemingly unresolvable ache.

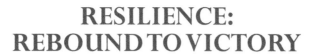

RESILIENCE:
REBOUND TO VICTORY

The year 2020 tested the enduring fortitude of the entire human species. The global pandemic impelled us to better understand and master the noble concept of resilience.

The words of the enigmatic American novelist Ernest Hemingway, taken out of context from his usually depressing tone, provide us with an uplifting introduction to a very timely exploration into the nature of resilience[63]:

> *"The world breaks everyone,*
>
> *and afterward,*
>
> *many are strong at the broken places."*

Without access to our current biological insights, Hemingway seemed to understand nature's intricate design that makes positive response to injury not only possible but highly successful. Our bodies are a thriving balance of breakdown and reconstruction.[64] We have an ingenious design, where teams of dedicated chemicals and cells destroy the old and broken while other teams follow them around rebuilding and rejuvenating. Even bone, the strongest of human tissue, is constantly being remodeled, adapting to physical stress to optimize its performance.

It is well proven that the healing process often leaves the tissue that infiltrates an injured site stronger than it was before the insult. I'm sure this is true for our emotional and spiritual existence, too. Hemingway's quote reminds us of the tremendous power to be gained in healing, both physically and emotionally. As in the case of bone, we develop new strength to accommodate new stresses and pressures, and this local strength often exceeds anything we had before.

Although the strength of a physical scar is greater than the surrounding, non-traumatized tissue, this contrast creates a new problem. The non-elasticity of physical scar tissue places greater stress on the surrounding muscle, ligament, and bone, leaving them at greater risk of subsequent injury. One of the objectives of physical therapy is to reduce the rigidity of scar tissue, just as one of the objectives of psychotherapy is to "soften" psychic scars to ensure more healthy psychodynamics after injury—in other words, to create resilience.

Resilience is a topic of much interest to both social scientists and growth seekers, for good reason. It drives two outcomes we care about: happiness and success. Happy people bounce back with smiles. Successful people roll with the punches, getting up quickly to continue their journeys.

But here is the terrifying observation lurking in Hemingway's quote: Not everybody gets stronger after facing adversity.

Not all *respond positively to injury.*

Not all *come back stronger.*

Not all *get back up.*

Not all *keep moving forward.*

So what drives our ability to respond with resilience? How can we be sure to be in the group that returns stronger after injury?

Our inquiry should be inspired by the powerful insight of the well-known human rights champion Nelson Mandela, who touched lives around the world with his iconic fortitude in the face of massive personal hardship[65]:

"Do not judge me by my successes;

judge me by how many times I fell down

and got back up again."

The reality is that levels of resilience vary between individuals. Some have it in abundance and keep bouncing back, all the way up the ladder, while others seem to wither at the first setback. Resilience can even fluctuate over time in the same person, as I'm sure each one of us can attest to, and can vary between different domains. For example, you may bounce back quickly at work but struggle in your personal life.

Why?

First, we must understand that resilience itself is a behavior, not an attribute. It's the outcome of a number of mindsets. Like the symptoms of a disease, we're better off understanding the underlying cause. It doesn't work to just say to someone, "Be more resilient." Resilience isn't something that can be turned on, like flipping a switch. Instead, we need to look behind the scenes to understand what drives resilience and build on it from there.

In our physical bodies, we have the opposing forces of degeneration and rejuvenation at work all the time. This is no different in our mental and emotional domains. Just as your physical body has two armies at work—one destroying and one building—so too does your mental and emotional being.[66]

And the default is degeneration. If we do nothing else, life breaks us down.

So, we must actively drive mental and emotional rejuvenation if we want to be resilient. Just as we pursue exercise, caloric balance, and good sleep to drive physical rejuvenation at the cellular, chemical, and even genetic levels, so we must find and feed the mental and emotional "builders" within.

There are six methods we can use to feed those mental and emotional builders:

1. *Having a neutral emotional response to setback enables rapid recovery.*
   You won't often find me recommending that you disengage emotionally.
   Most of the time I advocate strongly for the value of emotional
   engagement. But think about the way that your body copes with injury.
   If your immune and inflammatory cells went into mourning when you
   sustained a minor laceration, you might never heal. Instead, without
   hesitation, your body sends in the cells of rejuvenation to repair your
   injured tissue. We should emulate this in our lives. Get over setbacks fast
   and heal. Like your bones, your mind will remodel to cope with the new
   stress or circumstances that could otherwise derail you.

2. *Second, embrace your vulnerability. We're not always right in our*
   attitudes and planning. Things go wrong, and that's okay. Be vulnerable.
   Mistakes and setbacks are loaded with learning. Embrace both, and
   bounce back stronger.

3. *Yield to forces greater than you. I call this the art of situational yield.*
   As we get older, our bones become harder. While this may seem like
   an advantage, it is actually a disadvantage when we encounter trauma

because hard bones are more brittle. Instead of yielding to the stress, they fracture. While embracing an overall determination and unwillingness to give up in our day-to-day lives, it is vital to recognize where yielding protects you and preserves your strength for more important matters. Don't make your next heroic act your last.

4. *Your psyche thrives on thinking positive thoughts. Feed it. Actively engage in the proliferation of positive thoughts on an ongoing basis to nourish your capacity for resilience—every day, before you need it.*

5. *Sleep is the physical mode in which mental and emotional rejuvenation occurs. Many ambitious people believe that they can repair and refuel on the go. This is patently untrue. We are built to recover while we sleep, and sleep debt reduces your resilience significantly. While you sleep, you feed and nourish the army of good. So, sleep and rest.*

6. *Build an external environment that favors resilience. There is strong evidence that we have become more fragile and less resilient as we have moved away from tribal cultures toward more insular, independent lives. We need to actively maintain those close relationships that support and stimulate mental and emotional recoil. Positivity is mirrored. Surround yourself with supportive family and friends who give you energy and enhance your propensity for resilience.*

We are the architects of both our internal and our external environments. Smart design in both arenas enables resilience, which drives success, a concept well known to beloved American football coach and sporting legend Vince Lombardi, who said[67]:

"It's not whether you get knocked down:

it's whether you get up."

Working to build your capacity for resilience is only half of the battle, though. You also need to immunize yourself against resilience's deeply destructive enemy: helplessness.

Helplessness is the inability or unwillingness to pick yourself up from the floor, dust yourself off, and get on with life after a fall. Martin Seligman, distinguished professor of psychology at the University of Pennsylvania and founder of the Positive Psychology movement, spearheaded our current understanding of helplessness.

Seligman and his colleagues identified a state he termed "learned helplessness."[68] In this condition, the subject habitually acts helpless under duress. In early experiments, his laboratory dogs literally lay down in response to what they perceived to be overwhelming circumstances. You may have felt this way at the end of a hard week full of setbacks that tested your resilience.

When he delved further, Seligman found that helplessness is often the result of experiencing circumstances in which we are taught that our own efforts are meaningless.

Whether at home, or in school, or at work (or all three), when we are taught that our actions are of no consequence, we become helpless. Imagine the young child who tries to win the approval of a parent or teacher by working hard at school. But, regardless of their efforts, their parent or teacher focuses on the questions that the child got wrong or the talent of the children who got better grades. This child learns that their actions have no impact on the desired outcome (affirmation from the parent or teacher). There is grave risk of this young person developing learned helplessness.

Rather than bouncing back after a particularly hard exam, they may lie down and give up.

This situation is extremely dangerous because we are at risk of extrapolating our helplessness to other situations. Some personalities, especially those with more pessimistic tendencies, are likely to allow this helplessness, which began as a specific reaction to a particular circumstance, to extend into other functional domains. They begin to feel that their actions are meaningless across a broad range of important issues.

Of course, the opposite is true, too. Children who are taught that their actions are meaningful, especially those who are optimistic by nature, grow in confidence and resilience. It is easy to see how this becomes a virtuous cycle and how resilience becomes a major contributor to success.

But let's return to the helpless for a minute.

Seligman and his colleagues were not content to rest after discovering learned helplessness. They also wanted to know if it could be alleviated.[69]

In a fascinating array of experiments, they were able to show that both animals and people could be retrained to believe that their thoughts and actions mattered.[70] Through a variety of techniques that became the foundations of Positive Psychology, these pioneers demonstrated that we could systematically unlearn helplessness.[71]

As we diminish learned helplessness, what arises in its place are optimism, hopefulness, a belief that life's problems are surmountable, and a resilience that enables newfound success.

And that's not all: Seligman and his team were able to demonstrate that you can teach hopefulness.[72]

By teaching young animals and humans that their actions were meaningful, they were able to build lifelong resilience. Seligman called this phenomenon "immunization" against helplessness.[73] When they encountered unpredicted setbacks later in life, those who had been "immunized" were more resilient than their peers who had not received this training.

What does all this mean for you?

Doubt, fear, pessimism, and helplessness are products of our primitive, reptilian brain. To counteract those negative forces, we must use our cognitive brain to drive optimism and resilience. We can think our way to success, if we choose. We can confront negativity using the following five steps:

1. Recognize *the automatic negative thoughts when you meet resistance.*

2. Dispute *the negative thoughts using objective arguments. Your explanations about helplessness are seldom correct.*

3. Replace *these helpless thoughts with different explanations. Rather than telling yourself that you were knocked down because you are weak (and therefore helpless), explain to yourself that your opponent struck a well-timed, powerful blow. Remain hopeful in your ability to recover.*

4. Distract *yourself from negative thoughts. Recognize when you brood and hold onto helpless explanations. Action is a great distraction.*

5. *Over time, with patience and diligence, you will recognize the common negative assumptions you hold that precipitate helplessness.* Challenge *those assumptions at every opportunity, to fend off helplessness even before it presents itself.*

As always, life is a journey. None of this progress will happen overnight. I hope that the insight and pointers I've presented here will help you to fortify your own resilience.

Rocky Balboa, the come-back hero from the well-known Hollywood glory movie of the same name summarized his life philosophy, learned in the blood and sweat of the boxing ring, as follows[74]:

"It ain't about how hard you hit.

It's about how hard you can get hit and keep moving forward.

How much you can take, and keep moving forward."

Note: If you are experiencing severe helplessness, anxiety, depression, or suicidal thoughts, please seek out professional help. In particular, look for someone who understands Positive Psychology and cognitive therapy. These are powerful interventions, and there is every reason to believe that you will get an excellent result.

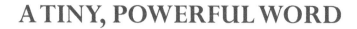

A TINY, POWERFUL WORD

My wife Karen was a schoolteacher. Every day, she worked with children striving to be the best that they could be. Through her work, she acquired a deep respect for the power of belief and an awareness of the danger of self-imposed mental limits. We human beings build dense boundaries for our own performance, usually within our own minds. This is the danger of our inner critic.

One thing I learned from Karen (actually, there are many wonderful things I learned from her) was the power of this tiny little word:

YET

If you use this word at the end of a phrase, you convert a damning sentence into one filled with promise and hope.

> *Try it:*
>
> *"I can't do math…yet."*
>
> *"I don't like chemistry…yet."*
>
> *"I can't lose weight…yet."*
>
> *"I'm not healthy…yet."*
>
> *"I haven't found happiness…yet."*
>
> *"I am not successful…yet."*
>
> *"Prosperity obviously isn't for me…yet."*

It's not just that the sentence sounds better when you add this tiny, powerful word. It's that, the more you say it, the more the phrase becomes self-fulfilling, and the more it describes a desirable *and attainable* future state. Over time, you convert your limitation into powerful self-belief. You will work and wait patiently for the promise you have made yourself. In the end, it *will* come true.

If you're struggling with the giant leap to prosperity or the long journey to abundance, be honest with yourself, but articulate this as a statement filled with hope. Complete your descriptive sentences with the tiny, powerful YET.

Then get back to work on the success you so richly desire and deserve.

RELATIONSHIP WITH OTHERS

SPREAD LOVE AND JOY, EFFORTLESSLY

A while back, I walked into the lobby of a hotel that was serving as the headquarters for a major national youth sports competition. Athletes from all over the USA (and a few individuals from other countries) had assembled for the biggest water polo tournament in the world: USA Water Polo's Junior Olympics.[75] The mood was infectious. Children and adults alike were walking around with big grins on their faces, proud and happy to be there. If you'd walked into the hotel as a total stranger, you couldn't help but have left with a smile!

The diffusion of positive mood was palpable, readily evident in the voices and actions of the hundreds of young aquatic athletes in the lobby and meeting rooms.

It was no accident that the hotel staff were friendlier than usual, too. They had been infected by the organic spread of positive energy. Frankly, I was sure that I could see taxi and bus drivers leaving the hotel with happy faces. I am convinced that their subsequent passengers also "caught" a little dose of the emotional gold flowing out of this glowing epicenter.

It is well known, both by observation and by scientific research, that mood is contagious, spreading *between* individuals.[76] What interests me most, though, is the internal chemistry that reinforces and escalates this emotional epidemic, because mood is also contagious *within* our own personal space.

The term *mood congruence* is used to describe mood's relationship with both perception and memory.[77] Your mood influences your perceptions of external stimuli. If you're feeling happy, you notice other happy sights and sounds with greater intensity than you do sad ones. At the same time, you somehow recall more joyful memories than you do sad ones.

These two phenomena tend to make mood self-reinforcing. Sadly, the same is true for negative mood, which sometimes has far-reaching negative consequences. But let's stay focused on the positive.

As each individual becomes a radiating center of positive affect, they infect those around them. This is what I term *mood diffusion*.

So, each of us has a choice in the role we play in society. We can choose how to affect the energy of our surroundings. We can choose to give energy or to withdraw it—and both will have far-reaching consequences. Choose wisely!

THE BEST
EXERCISE ADVICE EVER

What if I taught you a single exercise that worked more than 20 muscles and improved your health and happiness? What if I told you that you could do it anywhere, anytime; that it wouldn't cost a cent; and that it would benefit those around you? What if I told you that those who do it with the greatest intensity are rewarded with the longest lives?

You might be surprised to learn that the face is a highly mobile body part housing 43 muscles.[78] Scientists refer to these muscles as the "muscles of facial expression" because that is their job.[79] They twist, tweak, and contort our faces so that we can engage in nonverbal communication.

In theory, if you were to do the math on the number of unique facial gestures each of us could make, the figure would be an astounding 8.8 trillion! That is 8.8 followed by 12 zeros. With a global population of about 8 billion humans, this means that I would have over 1,000 unique facial expressions to share with each person on the planet. Or, I could use more than 300 million new expressions every day of my life. Whew! For all intents and purposes, we have an infinite range of facial expressions.

In practice, even if we could coordinate our faces well enough to execute all these gestures, our eyes and brains are not sophisticated enough to interpret each discrete nuance. Instead, scientists and computers are able to decipher 21 unique, consistently differentiable categories of facial gesture.[80] We can break these down further to six major emotions: happiness, sadness, surprise, fear, anger, and disgust (and some researchers add contempt as a seventh). The reason we get 21 categories out of these emotions is that some are compounded. For example, your face can show that you are happily surprised or sadly surprised. It is this nuanced communication repertoire that makes our faces such rich communication tools.

Of all these expressions, one stands out as having astonishing benefits for us: the simple smile.

Of course, the "simple" smile comes in a very wide variety of discretely recognizable versions: the beam, the shy smile, the smug smirk, the naughty grin, and many more. They are all good for you—even a fake smile, although it's only half as good as an authentic smile.

How does this fundamental expression of happiness benefit us? Let's start with how it benefits *others*. Smiling is contagious. Research has proven, beyond doubt, that seeing a smile induces others to smile.[81] This is as true with family and friends as it is with perfect strangers. In fact, the power of this life force is so strong that photographs of smiling faces are enough to evoke happiness in their viewers. This means that, each time you smile at somebody else, you give them the list of benefits below that you also enjoy for yourself.

When you exercise your 20-plus smiling muscles in beautiful harmony, this is how you (and the ones you smile at) benefit:

1. Better cardiovascular health. *Smiling reduces blood pressure, which contributes to a decrease in heart disease.[82]*

2. Reduced stress. *Smiling releases dopamine, endorphins, and the feel-good hormone serotonin, which enhance mood and reduce the adverse effects of stress.[83]*

3. Enhanced mood. *Independent of the above, the act of smiling makes you happy. As far back as 1872, Charles Darwin, in his book titled The Expression of the Emotions in Man and Animals, was the first scientist to recognize that "even the simulation of an emotion tends to arouse it in our minds."[84] Modern researchers know this as the "facial feedback hypothesis."[85] It is much easier to control our muscles than our emotions, so smiling is a simple way to brighten our mood.*

4. Enhanced attractiveness. *Research has shown many times over that a smiling face is more attractive to others than a non-smiling face.[86] Whether you're trying to find a mate, work well with colleagues, or simply live more easily, smiling works.*

5. Better relationships. *People who smile more have more stable and satisfying marriages and long-term relationships.[87]*

6. Improved longevity. *This is the ultimate evidence for the value of smiling. In a landmark study published in 2010 in the Journal of the Association for Psychological Science[88], researchers demonstrated how those who flashed authentic smiles lived longer than fake-smilers who lived longer than non-smilers.*

You might argue that we're living through times in which it is difficult to smile. But now, more than ever, it's imperative that we *do* smile. How many problems could be solved and how much better would we be able to work together if we just smiled at one another? Not only is it good for "them"; it has profound value for "us," too.

Here, then, is my prescription for the most important exercise you will ever do:

- *Speak face to face, using a video chat program rather than the telephone when you can't meet in person. Smile while talking.*

- *Walk into your child's bedroom to talk (and smile) rather than sending a text message.*

- *Walk into your colleague's office to talk (and smile) rather than sending an email.*

- *Use emojis if you text or, even better, use Snapchat. A smile without words is more valuable than words without a smile.*

- *Smile, smile, and smile some more. Smile spontaneously, warmly, sincerely, and generously, for yourself and for others!*

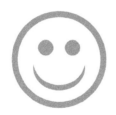

LAUGHTER:
A HEALTHY CONTAGION

Close your eyes and picture a happy gathering. Visualize the faces of friends and family. Close your eyes tighter now, squeezing out all other senses except sound. Hear the noises of the happiness. I'd be very surprised if laughter wasn't there, possibly even the dominant sound—and for good reason: Laughter drives health and happiness.

"When the first baby laughed for the first time,

the laugh broke into a thousand pieces

and they all went skipping about,

and that was the beginning of fairies."

~ J.M. Barrie[89]

As we begin to interact with the world as tiny infants, we watch and copy those around us. Before our brain develops the connections that enable speech, we learn to smile and laugh.[90] This is a curious phenomenon that emphasizes the value of an immensely powerful act. You might question why babies should choose to copy something that adults do with much lower frequency than children. Actually, it's not so surprising. Adults laugh far more in the presence of babies than they do elsewhere, underlining the deep association between this instinctive reflex and true happiness.[91]

True laughter is a spontaneous gesture that is triggered unconsciously. It cannot be forced, making it a hard subject for scientists to study. We know that the average adult laughs 18 times a day.[92] The vast majority of times, it's not in response to a joke, indicating that it's less an expression of humor than an expression of comfort and familiarity (and sometimes even nervousness). We laugh much more when we are with other people, reinforcing the role of laughter in interpersonal bonding, a profoundly healthy engagement.[93]

Laughter appears to have several physical benefits for us, including a decrease in blood pressure, an increase in blood flow, and an increase in oxygenation of the blood.[94] It also recruits activity from the facial, core, and respiratory muscles; in fact, it is estimated that 100 laughs are equivalent to 15 minutes on an exercise bicycle.[95]

Laughter has been shown to increase the number and activity of potent immune cells that are involved with attacking foreign pathogens (infections) and cancer.[96] It also boosts other critical cells that are responsible for antibody production.[97] These benefits may all be related to the laughter-induced decrease in stress hormones—those chemicals that, if left unchecked, can suppress the immune system, increase blood pressure, and increase the number of clotting cells in the blood (predisposing us to heart attack and stroke).[98] Laughter also releases dopamine, endorphins, and the feel-good hormone serotonin to enhance mood and further reduce the adverse effects of stress.[99]

Like smiling, laughter is contagious, as anybody who "gets the giggles" knows. So, when we laugh with friends, we not only benefit personally, but we share the health and happiness with them, too.

I have often found it sad that we laugh less as adults than we did as children. It seems that, once we get "serious" about life, we cannot be seen to be trivial or frivolous. If only we could remember that laughter is great medicine.

So, whether you're an overworked business leader, an exhausted parent, or simply taking a well-earned break from back-to-back meetings, stop…take a deep breath…and laugh out loud!

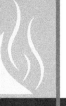

VULNERABILITY:
A SURPRISING STRENGTH

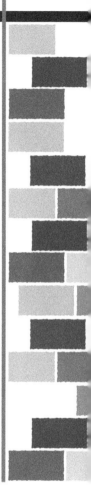

During one of our regular beach walks a few years back, my wife and I paused to watch the 2017 World Adaptive Surfing Championships.[100] In this sport, so-called "disabled" athletes deny their physical limits, competing for international medals.

Watching these acts of great courage and persistence brought tears to my eyes, and one moment in particular caught my attention.

A young man in his mid-20s was preparing to surf in the championship heat. He had been left paralyzed below the waist following a horrific car accident. His flaccid legs simply wouldn't respond to any messages from his brain asking them to support or move him.

His coach bent over and scooped him up like a child to carry him into the water.

I wasn't sure how I'd feel to be this young man. But I know that I would probably struggle with a deep sense of inadequacy at having to be carried.

How sad—not for him, but for me!

Far from my piteous response, this young hero had embraced his vulnerability, graciously accepting the loving help of his coach.

Through his "weakness," he was strong.

Human history is filled with stories that capture the intimate juxtaposition of vulnerability and strength.

A hero is frequently born from a character who hits rock bottom. Urban legend has it that successful entrepreneurs must experience bankruptcy before they enjoy success. The mythological phoenix flies up from the ashes of its predecessor, rising with new life. Out of war comes peace.

Vulnerability is a powerful seed for rebirth and growth.

In both her scholarly and her popular writing, resilience expert Brené Brown[101] highlights the value of the "face-plant," that moment in which we find ourselves face down in the arena of life. She guides her followers on how to respond to this situation, suggesting that, when we embrace vulnerability, and even seek it out, we open the door for profound, transformational growth.

Without accepting his vulnerability, this elite athlete wouldn't have been competing at the highest level, and he wouldn't be wearing the gold medal and the champion's title that is rightfully his today.

In contrast, how often has "strength" been my own weakness? How many victories have I denied myself by hiding behind false strength or frail ego, instead of asking for and accepting help?

How many victories have you denied yourself the exact same way?

Challenge yourself to explore your own vulnerability.

When we are truly vulnerable, we engage in powerful actions that fuel growth. We *listen*, *ask* for help, *yield* to insurmountable challenges, and above all *invite* rebirth.

When you embrace your vulnerability, you, too, will be a champion.

THE MANY FACES
OF EMPATHY

Angus was nervous. It was our first meeting, and he shifted restlessly in his seat through our introductions.

He was a high achiever. He'd sailed through his undergraduate studies on a full scholarship and been recruited to a leading medical school, where he earned recognition for clinical competence and academic leadership. He'd accepted a top fellowship and was working hard, enhancing his reputation amongst peers and patients as a caring physician.

But that day was different. That day, he was struggling with a big question. He was no longer sure that he was on the right professional pathway. His uncertainty seemed to be growing daily. He lay awake at night consumed by anxiety. Having been so sure for so long, doubt had now brought him to the point of despair.

Halfway through our first meeting, we uncovered a phenomenon that deeply colored his life, had informed his early career decisions, and would clearly be important in the big decision he now faced.

This powerful insight emerged as we discussed his clinical practice. He recounted the emotions that surfaced when he helped his sickest patients.

His strong blue eyes filled with tears as he told me, "I feel their pain so intensely, Roddy, that sometimes I just have to look away."

In this simple, powerful phrase, he revealed how profoundly his life was governed by empathy.

Empathy is one of Mother Nature's greatest gifts, which enables us to build profound relationships within our respective social groups. It is the primal glue that holds us together. When we deeply experience the joy and pain of those we love and live with, we build indestructible bonds that ensure our survival as individuals, as a tribe, and as a species.

And scientists know a lot about empathy. We know where it resides in the human brain and the many associated centers of higher function that integrate it into our modern life.[102] We understand how brain injury can disrupt it, and we know how emotional trauma can affect it.[103]

And we also know that the impact empathy has isn't always positive. In fact, it poses very real danger to human society. Many prominent researchers identify it as the root cause of political and racial polarization—something we see all too much of today.[104]

You see, empathy is at the root of the "us versus them" phenomenon.

It selectively reinforces intense bonds between close social allies, sometimes leaving "them" (anybody else) on the outside. "They" then become the object of *reverse empathy*. Instead of love, trust, and harmony, reverse empathy leads to hatred, mistrust, and hostility. We're seeing these sad consequences spilling out in all sorts of ugly social and political expressions both nationally and globally.

But let's get back to the science of empathy.

Empathy alone doesn't drive our choices and behavior. For this to happen, we need its close cousin *compassion*.

It is compassion that converts empathetic feelings into action. This is the difference between the many who walk past the destitute homeless man sleeping in the gutter and the few good Samaritans who actively reach out to offer him meaningful help.

Incidentally, this attenuation also holds true for the activation of reverse empathy. For both the good and the bad outcomes, feelings need to be translated into action, and only a few are inspired to convert hostile feelings into actions of hatred.

So, both individually and collectively, we need to work carefully to balance the upsides and downsides of empathy in order to benefit from Mother Nature's great gift.

At the macro-societal level, we need to understand that love for self and family puts us at risk of alienating "them." We need to understand how detrimental this can be as it comes back to threaten the sanctity of "us." We need to foster in our children, through our own examples, the urgent need to understand and love both "us" and "them." If we fail in this, one of Mother Nature's greatest gifts will become our greatest downfall.

Now let's get back to Angus.

I know that empathy will be a constant and pervasive theme as we continue to explore his individual future.

On the one hand, I know that this powerful gift has driven him to choose a caring profession. He has followed the voice that deeply understands the condition of his patients. This is the upside, and both he and his patients are rewarded for his gift.

On the other hand, I have little doubt that we will soon discover that his empathy has also exaggerated the influence of the well-intended thoughts and desires of teachers, friends, and family on his early decisions. I am sure that his career choice has been influenced by a desire to appease *their* hopes and aspirations, too. So, empathy has also become a prominent source of the immense pain he feels as he approaches his vocational crisis.

Angus must carefully pick a path between these two powerful empathetic forces in order to reach the fulfillment and happiness he deserves. Once he is clear on the healthy direction in which his empathy should lead him, he will again stride forward in confidence and joy.

I'm curious to see where the fresh insight takes him on his magnificent journey.

I hope that you, like Angus, will have the courage to look within, where magic happens and dreams come to life. I hope that you will explore the powerful role that empathy has played in bringing you to where you are today and, more importantly, how it can empower you further to reach the success you so richly desire and deserve.

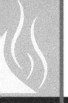

THE POWER
OF AFFIRMATION

It was late. The wintry sun had long since disappeared for its well-earned rest, while the full moon had started her journey across the night sky, peeking over the mountaintops in the distance. The lights in my office cast a warm beam on the snowy landscape outside. Across the way, through the bony fingers of leafless trees, I saw the lights of the hospital twinkling. I hoped that my patients would rest quietly, soaking in the moon's healing power on this beautiful night.

I often worked late. I cared deeply about my patients and spent the last hour of each day checking their lab results and progress reports before preparing for those I would see the next day.

Happy that all was complete, and ready for the morning, I packed my bags. Grabbing my coat from behind the door, I headed for the main lobby and made the short walk to the parking garage. I was excited to get home to my wife and young children. Passing through the door into the cold garage, I saw the kind face of Andreas. He was the security guard who watched over the main entrance through the dark and lonely nights.

Tonight, his eyes sparkled.

I stopped to greet him and to hear the latest news about his youngest grandchild. Gesturing me to wait, he disappeared into the back office, and I could hear him furiously opening desk drawers. He emerged clutching a well-handled piece of paper and rushed toward me, thrusting the page into my hands.

In the dim light, I read the short paragraph addressed to him. It came from the head of the hospital. It was written in simple, direct language, thanking him for his exemplary contribution to the welfare of our community. It praised him for his unselfish dedication to his unseen vigil, appreciating the many long, dark hours that he spent alone keeping our offices and our patients' records safe.

As I finished reading, I looked up at his beaming face. I confess that it brought a tear to my tired eyes. Before I turned to walk to my car, I shook his hand. He held my grip and my gaze for a few seconds and in his old, gruff voice said, "You know, Doc, this letter will feed me for years."

In our brief exchange, two dedicated, hard-working colleagues doing their best to make the world a better place had shared a profound truth. Andreas' colorful expression had crisply captured for me the immense power of affirmation. It remains at the core of all my teaching and coaching. It's a simple, natural way to unlock the very best in ourselves and each other.

So, whether you write a short note or take a few extra moments to say a simple "thank you," remember that you can feed another's soul in the best possible way through the power of affirmation.

PARTNERS AND PARENTING

NOURISH YOUR FIRE
WITH CARE

Our core vitality is like a fire.

At times, we enjoy the dynamic warmth and energy of a robust blaze within us. I'm sure you've experienced wild days where your internal fire seems to surge, out of control, a powerful mix of exuberance and chaos.

At other times, our flames may dwindle, leaving only glowing cinders that we can hopefully resuscitate. Perhaps right now you feel you have nothing left but embers, needing to be carefully brought back to a full flame.

Each of us is responsible for tending to our own fire. This careful oversight of our vital energy is just like the delicate, nuanced supervision we employ in nurturing a real fire.

If you're lucky, you'll have people in your life who invite you to help in nurturing their fires.

As a spouse or partner, you have the unique privilege of helping to guard and nourish the other's flame.

We parents also get to nurture the flames of our offspring.

Many of us, in enthusiasm and love, rush around looking for wood to pile onto our own and each other's fires. For some reason, we are especially enthusiastic about piling logs onto our children's fires.

Our fervent desire to see a massive, roaring bonfire has us heaping on more wood at every opportunity, with significant negative consequences.

Instead of blindly feeding the fire, I invite you to read and remember this beautiful little poem written by Judy Brown, an educational leader, author, and poet.[105] I carry it with me always, a simple reminder that sometimes doing less is more, especially as a parent.

FIRE

What makes a fire burn
is space between the logs,
a breathing space.
Too much of a good thing,
too many logs
packed in too tight
can douse the flames
almost as surely
as a pail of water would.
So building fires
requires attention
to the spaces in between,
as much as to the wood.
When we are able to build
open spaces
in the same way
we have learned
to pile on the logs,
then we can come to see how
it is fuel, and absence of the fuel
together, that make fire possible.
We only need to lay a log
lightly from time to time.
A fire
grows
simply because the space is there,
with openings
in which the flame
that knows just how it wants to burn
can find its way.

Keeping your flame burning brightly takes special care and attention. Act wisely and purposefully—and sometimes act less—as you nurture the fire that drives your own success.

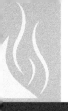

RESOLVING RELATIONSHIP CONFLICT, AUTHENTICALLY

Relationships require hard work.

Biology takes care of the short term; hormones drive infatuation in the early days. After that, we all must work to stay in love. Why?

Surprisingly, that answer comes from biology, too.

You see, we humans are not simple beings. In fact, we're fascinatingly complex mosaics. Our evolutionary success is driven by our enormously sophisticated and versatile brain that has the capacity to present us to the world in a broad range of ways. We're like a giant, living Swiss Army knife: the most advanced multitool on the planet. And our brain is the supercomputer that drives this within-person diversity.

Think about yourself for a moment. Like everyone else, you're a kind, calm, thoughtful, reasonable, and caring human being. But if you're honest with yourself, there are moments when you're really not this wonderful person I just described. In fact, there are probably moments when you're far from them!

There are times that you fly into a blind rage or withdraw into almost total silence in sadness or unhappiness. There are times when you're overcome by jealousy or fear, and a completely different *you* emerges.

In truth, you have many faces. One person, many faces, each driven from the single brain you were born with.

I'm not talking about multiple personalities. I'm talking about the many ways that you've learned to behave—each so discretely powerful that you sometimes appear to be many people within one human frame.

Each different *you* results from a collection of nerve centers in your brain that fire together to produce a discrete attitude or behavior set.[106] Repeated collective activation of these pathways induces them to form dense "maps" in your brain that represent the range of sub-personalities that lead you in your day-to-day life. And all these sub-personalities are good. Each uniquely mapped sub-personality is specialized for a different situation, and each behavior set that results from its activation is so discrete that you may look (and feel) like an entirely different person under its influence. It's a magnificent design that enables your survival and success.

But here is the problem: As you reinforce these psychobiological entities, they often become dominant—even default—players that very willingly step up to lead, especially in stressful situations. And some of these good players tend to become not-so-good players in their deep commitment to serving you.

These not-so-good players are seriously committed to protecting you. Their job is to help you survive, and they selfishly take care of your safety first, putting everything and everyone else into a distant second place.

We usually don't like these not-so-good parts of ourselves; they can be downright nasty, they tend to get us into trouble, and they are highly active in relationship disputes. But they are very real!

In times of distress, they rise up to the surface in a spontaneous and determined protective effort—and since only one of your parts can be leading at any one time, your kind and loving parts move below the radar and into the background.

At such times, you're not necessarily the nicest person to be around. And when your and your partner's not-so-good parts are leading at the same time...well, it's certainly not a recipe for a harmonious relationship!

Sadly, the statistics are not encouraging. Mathematically, if you had only two parts—a good one and a not-so-good one—you would enjoy only one out of every four days in harmony with your life partner. And if you had four not-so-good parts (and most of us have many more), this success would be dramatically reduced. Without any overriding self-control, you might enjoy only one good day together each month!

But there is good news.

Each of these not-so-good parts can be controlled by the very same mind that drives the beautiful you—the authentic *you*, the authentic self you were born with, the beautiful, calm, kind, caring, confident, trusting SELF that is the best part of you.

Since your brain, like every other organ, works for you—well, at least, it *should* work for you—you are able to decide which part of your brain takes the lead at any moment and in any situation.

When your authentic SELF leads, life is good. And it's even better when your and your partner's authentic SELVES show themselves at the same time. Then, you are able to enjoy a loving and fulfilling relationship.

With courage, patience, skilled insight, and training, you can increase the likelihood of putting your authentic SELF in control, even in times of distress.

So, when you find yourself in the middle of a hot marital argument, don't say, "You're ruining my life because you're always jealous (or angry, or sad, or afraid)!" Instead, identify calmly that, "A part of you is jealous (or angry, or sad, or afraid) right now," and then insist on speaking with the person you love, the authentic self of your partner that has been pushed aside by their protective part.

And, if you're the one feeling jealous (or angry, or sad, or afraid), then calmly state that, "A part of me is feeling jealous (or angry, or sad, or afraid)." You will notice that, as you call attention to this not-so-good part and explicitly state that those not-so-good emotions and behaviors belong to that part—and not your authentic SELF—you create a kaleidoscope of uplifting possibilities.

Without those possibilities, your partner had to somehow negotiate harmony with your not-so-good parts—not an easy or a pleasant task. But now, instead, you and your partner can work with the not-so-good part rearing its ugly head, asking it to step aside so that you can again deal directly with the one whom you fell in love with. And, together, when both of your authentic SELVES lead, you will solve any problem with ease.

When you perfect this approach, you stand a much better chance of achieving a harmonious, productive relationship that will last a lifetime. You see, the beauty of this magnificent brain design is that the parts of your brain that you nourish will flourish. As you work to keep each mapped sub-personality performing its *good* role, and limiting its *not-so-good* influence, you fundamentally alter the structure and function of your brain, rewiring it for good!

I hope that you will have the courage to explore your inner world, either alone or with your life partner, and see that this pathway to a balanced and integrated life will lead to loving and rewarding partnerships.

THE RARE ART
OF A GOOD APOLOGY

One rainy day, Harvard Business School researchers[107] sent a student into a train station to ask commuters if he could borrow their cell phones. With half the people, he made a direct request, without any preemptive softening. With the other half, he started by apologizing for the rain before asking to borrow the stranger's phone.

The superfluous apology (after all, the rain was hardly the student's fault) made strangers five times more likely to trust him with their phone—a graphic demonstration of the value of empathy and the power of a simple apology.

In the most comprehensive study to date, social scientists from Ohio State University[108] ranked the importance of six elements of an apology. They found that effective apologies contained most, if not all, of these elements.

The most important element is to *acknowledge responsibility* (as when saying, "I made a mistake" *and* "It's my fault").

The next most powerful element is to *offer to repair* the situation. Most of us understand that words are cheap, so, when your actions back up your words, people believe you are truly sorry.

In this study, *expressions of regret* and *declarations of repentance* were both important, followed by *explanations for what went wrong* (although many practiced communicators will warn that explanations may erode the perceived sincerity of your apology).

It turns out that the least valuable element is to *request forgiveness*...but it won't do you any harm, either!

You may now be tempted to carefully plan your next apology to include all of these basic elements. You may even rehearse what you'll say, determined to have the offended person hear your apology the way you intend it. But I believe that there is one key principle not explicitly identified in this research that you will find invaluable.

Have you ever wondered why people shout when they get angry or argue, or when they have been wronged?

The answer is confoundingly obvious: We raise our voices when we think we have not been heard.

So, I propose that the fundamental secret to a successful apology is to show the offended person that they have been heard.

I once overheard a beautiful conversation between a young mother and her angry toddler.

Actually, the little boy was beyond angry…he'd just thrown a major tantrum. He had opened his lunch box to find that his favorite snack was missing.

"I'm very angry!" he shouted.

"Why?" Mom asked quietly.

"Because I'm very hungry," he proclaimed.

"Is that all?" she politely probed.

"No. You left out the cheese!" he blurted.

"Is that all?" she questioned.

"No!" he pouted. "You always give John his favorites."

"Is that all?" she calmly inquired.

"No! I think you love him more than me!" he announced, the storm within him finally reaching its furious peak as he dissolved into tears.

At this point, she gently held his hands, looked into his eyes, apologized for forgetting his favorite snack, and assured him that she loved him every bit as much as she loved his brother.

The offended child (and the captivated onlookers) had no doubt at all that he had been heard. And life continued smoothly.

Is that all?

Try preceding your next apology with this powerful question, repeated as many times as necessary to get to the root of the issue. It will help you to probe the depth of the offended person's pain, setting you up for a meaningful apology— once they have been fully heard.

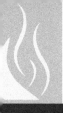

THE SCIENCE
OF COMPLIMENTS

A compliment is a powerful verbal gift.

I have written often about the power of giving and the tremendous value that this simple act unlocks for both the giver and the receiver. For the most part, I tend to emphasize the value for the giver. When we are generous, we honor our natural design and trigger deep biological responses that unlock health and happiness. Often, it is the least expensive gifts, like affirmation and praise, that evoke the most benefit. And most of us are very comfortable giving affirmation.

But how do you *receive* praise?

Many of us are uncomfortable when we get a compliment. At best, we reluctantly accept the kind words. At worst, we feel ashamed and unworthy of the praise.

Several factors drive our discomfort. Sometimes it's just downright embarrassing when somebody identifies our strong points publicly. Other times, we find the implied scrutiny uncomfortable; we feel exposed and self-conscious. Mainly, we have been raised by good parents who taught us humility, and we worry that readily accepting a compliment might be misinterpreted as conceit or arrogance.

But when we are incapable of accepting compliments, we starve ourselves of a vital and readily available nutrient.

Compliments are wonderful gifts, and we should learn to accept them openly, with warmth and gratitude, for four main reasons:

1. When we receive a gift, Mother Nature triggers the release of hormones like serotonin and dopamine that make us happy and healthy.[109]

2. Words of affirmation reinforce our self-belief, especially when they come from somebody we like and respect.[110] When we believe we are valuable, we become more valuable. Outside opinion is a powerful ally for our cognitive brain in its fight against the undermining voice of our primitive reptilian brain.

3. When we accept a compliment, we express gratitude, which itself is a powerful stimulant of health and happiness through well-recognized biological pathways.

4. Finally, when we openly acknowledge the sentiment and intent of kind words, we complete the circle of giving that starts deep in the emotional brain of the giver. In gaining from their words, we reward the giver. They too enjoy Mother Nature's magical design and are rewarded with health and happiness.

So when you get your next compliment, don't reject it stoically. Rather, look the giver in the eye, give them a huge, warm smile, and say a simple "thank you."

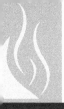

BALANCING WORK AND LIFE

How many times have you complained about not having a good work-life balance? The funny thing is, you hardly ever hear anyone complain about having too much life and too little work, making this a rather lopsided "imbalance."

I've mused on this topic often, usually when I've overburdened myself with work and left myself insufficient time to enjoy life, and I have a few ideas to share with you that I hope will be valuable on your own work-life journey.

To start, I have a question for you: How often do you drive in the middle of the road—precisely in the middle? Well, not really the middle of the road, but in the center of your lane?

Undoubtedly, you're a good driver, and your attention never wanders, and you've never been distracted by a conversation or a text message, so your answer to my question is, naturally, "always." You *always* drive in the middle of your lane.

But let's examine this a little closer.

Truth be told, you hardly ever drive exactly in the middle. You're almost always on one side or the other, shifting from being a little too far over to the left to being a little too far over to the right and back again.

Good drivers continuously and smoothly make minute adjustments, often subliminally, to correct their positions. Bad drivers, on the other hand, make wild lurches and swing their cars from side to side.

I've come to see work-life balance in the same way.

Just as it's rare to drive in the middle of the lane, you're seldom truly perfectly balanced between work and life. Instead, if you're managing things well, you're continuously, smoothly, and often subliminally making tiny adjustments to ensure that you're adequately balanced.

So what else can we learn from good drivers about how to master the work-life balance?

Good drivers know the areas that are dangerous, the places on either side of the lane where it is simply unsafe to drive. On one side, they run the risk of hitting oncoming traffic. On the other side, they run the risk of ending up in a ditch.

More than this, good drivers have two additional lines that they pay attention to; let's call them the "lines of tolerance." When they reach one of these two invisible lines, they realize it's time to take quick corrective action…before it's too late and they find themselves in the danger zone.

Experienced drivers don't stress about staying in their lane because they're subconsciously aware of and responsive to these invisible guiding lines that keep them far from oncoming traffic and the ditch.

Similarly, you needn't be stressed about your own work-life balance.

The trick is to define your danger zones and lines of tolerance, and simply correct before you get into big trouble.

I suggest that you be very deliberate about defining the lines of tolerance in your life. How many hours do you want to spend with your children, and partner, and hobbies? Is it okay to spend quality time with your family only in the morning or evening? What about your friends? Is once a year enough to see them? And how about your favorite pastimes? Is it sufficient to squeeze in five minutes for them once a week? Or do you want more? Choose your lines, and watch them closely.

Good drivers also concentrate on their driving. Once you've deliberately set your lines, periodically examine how you're doing. Over time, you'll learn to correct before you get into trouble. As with the good driver, deliberate attention to detail soon becomes second nature. Maintaining balance becomes easy and stress-free.

You can also count on your fellow travelers to help you. How often have you had to flash your lights or honk your horn to warn another driver that their attention is wavering? Or has your partner in the front seat next to you ever given you a gentle warning to return to your lane? Contract with your loved ones, friends, and colleagues to alert you when you're beyond your lines of tolerance.

Don't stress if you feel that you're out of balance. You're not alone; remember, we're all at least a little out of balance most of the time. Like the driver, we're seldom in the exact middle of the lane. Instead, we smoothly glide from one side to the other, finding an overall balance as we stay within our lines of tolerance.

Finally, if you're ever in doubt about a work-life decision, I recommend that you apply the rearview mirror test.

Imagine you're at the end of your journey, or at least well into your life's journey. You glance in the rearview mirror to see the history of your life receding behind you.

I know too many people who have looked back only to be shocked at how tiny the images of their children and loved ones appear. Instead of seeing friends and family occupying retrospective prominence, they are devastated to notice a giant commitment to work obscuring their view.

It's certainly not my place to tell you where to put your focus, or where to draw your own limits. But I do want to remind you that there will come a time when you can't go back. The decisions you make today profoundly affect what you'll see in your rearview mirror many years from now. And the images will become smaller and smaller as time passes.

Next time you're contemplating a decision that affects your work-life balance, take a quick look in the mirror. That should help you to get it right.

So drive confidently down the road of life, knowing that you have all the tools you need to create the perfect work-life balance for you!

HELP YOURSELF FIRST

It's a crazy suggestion. Yet all airlines advise us to put on our own oxygen masks before looking after our children. This is so contrary to every parenting instinct… but is it good advice?

I started thinking about this in the context of health and happiness.

Through my own life, there have been times when I was forced to choose between exercising and doing something with my children. And so, I often skipped exercise to be with them.

Actually, I always tried to do both. But, as you'll probably know from your own life, this isn't easy.

So, I often put my children first, ahead of my own health. That sounds like the right thing to do, doesn't it?

I now believe this is wrong.

Many years ago, in the midst of a highly successful high-profile career as a physician-scientist and corporate leader, I woke up to the fact that I was suffering from gross self-neglect.

In my sincere efforts and laudable determination to be a good husband and father, I was working long hours under very challenging circumstances to provide extremely well for my family. I was proud of this, and still am today. And, after traveling all week, I would come home to my family and pursue my devotion to my children with great enthusiasm and commitment. I took very good care of them and their needs, and I was proud of this, too.

But I was headed rapidly toward a quadruple bypass or similar physical disaster. Here I was, a physician and scientist who knew better than anyone else in the boardroom how to take care of myself.

And I wasn't doing it.

I simply didn't have the time to be an exceptional business leader and the world's best father and take care of myself. And so, I put my children first. And in doing so, I moved us all one small step closer to disaster.

Luckily, I realized it just in time.

When I started to prioritize my own healthy habits, I put myself in a better position to take care of my children. Instead of being incapacitated by my poor health and unhappiness, I had the strength and enthusiasm to care for them. Rather than being the exhausted couch potato who drags himself home at the end of the workday, or the gray-faced executive recovering from his first heart attack, I had energy and joy to invest in them.

More important still is the fact that I modeled healthy behavior for them. Through my unequivocal commitment to exercising regularly, balancing calories, sleeping well, and managing my stress, I modeled the behavior they need to pursue if they want to be healthy and happy for life—and that is my greatest wish for them.

Our children learn more from observing our behavior than they do from the words we speak. My children could see that I was healthy and happy. They witnessed the rewards of the transformation in my own life and have experienced the impact of my wellness in *their* lives. Today they thank me for putting my oxygen mask on first.

Next time you have a difficult choice like this, please consider that the "crazy" advice of the airlines may be appropriate and remember that taking care of yourself benefits those around you, too.

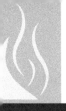

MY ROYAL PLEA
TO ALL PARENTS

Parents of young children often ask me what they should do to raise confident, successful young men and women. Here is what I tell them, based on my understanding of the neuroscience of the human brain and the power of belief:

Treat them like royals!

To help them understand further, I ask them to enter the theatre of their imagination and picture their children dressed as young members of a royal family on an important day. Picture them standing on a balcony overlooking a crowded square filled with adoring subjects. Picture them walking with their family among the crowd, heads high as they stride with a confident gait. Their faces, body language, and behavior ooze confidence. The world is theirs, and they can choose their own futures.

The human brain works in a wonderful way: If our brain is filled with positive thoughts that resonate with our emotional desires, belief flows easily and naturally. And this is the secret!

The royal child hears affirmation at every corner. The whole world shouts out, "You are worthy!" Their ears faithfully pass the message on to their brain, in particular to their cognitive brain. Their cognitive brain hears this message hour after hour, day after day. It becomes deeply ingrained in their being, and they believe—truly *believe*.

Because they believe, they walk tall and think big. They don't hear the nagging voice of their primitive brain urging caution as we do. Its paltry efforts are dwarfed by the resounding echoes in their cognitive brain: "You are worthy, you are worthy" becomes "I am worthy, I am worthy, *I am worthy*!" With this refrain, desires become belief, which become actions and success.

It's a simple recipe.

Now, most children don't have hordes of fans and an entourage sharing the constant affirmation that royals have. That's where we step in as parents. Our voices have to become the affirmation of the masses. Our voices have to shout loudly, every hour of every day, "You are worthy, you are worthy, you are worthy!" Our children's ears will faithfully pass the message on to their cognitive brains, and soon, belief becomes success.

I do have one word of caution: Even as you soak their growing brains in the "you are worthy" message, it must be balanced with the twin guidance that it is hard work that will be the forerunner of their success. Self-worthiness in the absence of hard work is *entitlement*, a dangerous affliction for royals and lesser mortals alike.

Finally, here is the most challenging part of this instruction for all parents: We have to model this royal behavior for our children. We have to model self-belief and self-worth.

Many parents are surprised to find, when they attend a parenting workshop based on the neuroscience of raising successful children, that we spend most of the time focusing on their own (the parents', that is) sense of self-worth. This is because children may or may not listen to our words, but they always notice, and usually follow, our actions—for better or for worse.

SIBLING RIVALRY: A HEALTHY FORCE OF NATURE

As far back as the legendary competition of Cain and Abel, siblings have competed for the love and attention of their parents. Generally, the competitive outbreaks are intermittent, contextualized by periods of love and affection; the rough times are mainly short lived and without major injury.

Regardless, whether gentle and infrequent or persistent and hostile, sibling rivalry is a puzzle to many of us.

In my work as an executive coach, I speak with many exasperated parents who feel guilty that their "poor" parenting skills allow such unattractive competitiveness. I propose instead that this rivalry is natural, healthy behavior that is better embraced and guided than regretted and suppressed.

Many instincts drive modern sibling rivalry. Birth order and developmental stage impact its expression; children compete to define who they are.[111] Older children may try to preserve the dominance they enjoy from early physical, emotional, and mental advantage. Conversely, younger children may rebel against older siblings, fighting for independent expression and a share of the family voice.

Also, children benefit from parental attention. When this is scarce, their instinct is to compete for the limited resources.[112] Our stressful lives can limit the availability of parental kindness and, at the same time, impede a child's ability to manage natural tensions without resorting to hostility.

How, then, do we as parents help make sibling rivalry a force for good?

Parental example is a powerful means of influencing rivalry behavior. Families that model tolerance and peace should not be surprised to find it in their children.

As parents, we should acknowledge and listen to each child's unique needs. Celebrate differences, praising each child loudly for their unique talents and achievements. Equal treatment is not appropriate, but equal attention, love, and praise are.

We should look for and reward good behavior and be prepared to model kind and peaceful ways to address and resolve conflicts.

We should try very hard not to compare our children with each other, including in subtle, non-obvious ways.[113] Rather than have them try to clean their rooms quicker than each other, have them race against the clock. Rather than rewarding the child who gets the highest grades, create incentives for any of your children who improve in a class. Don't get involved or pick sides. Even perpetuating a nickname that implies comparison, like "Speedy" or "Handsome," can be unintentionally harmful.

If you recognize that your own stress is exaggerating natural tensions, be kind to yourself. It takes courage to own this. Don't reproach yourself or describe your condition with harsh self-criticism. Take active steps to remediate, and celebrate the fact that each family has built-in stress detectors, like sibling rivalry, that are early warning systems. If you can, show your children that you understand how your impatience or distraction is part of the problem. Modeling this in an active way without letting shame detract from your important status within the family is an invaluable life lesson for all involved.

Your guidance during calm moments is more valuable than your desperate attempts to calm a violent outburst. Use happy times to discuss and model awareness and appreciation for different styles and personalities within the family.

Of course, dangerous or hurtful disputes must be stopped, ideally by diverting the energy toward more fruitful discussions. Decide if a conflict is harmful and, if not, either watch quietly as your children develop their own conflict-resolution skills or help them to negotiate toward a win-win situation.

Celebrate peace when it returns, and reward your children generously when they find their own path to a safe and mutually fruitful outcome.

I hope that this article helps you to appreciate the value of sibling rivalry and provides you with strategies for channeling it positively toward healthy growth for the entire family. Even as we guide the development of our children, we advance our own insight and strength as caring, engaged adults.

RAISING SUCCESSFUL CHILDREN

A few years ago, I participated in a wonderful conference attended by a group of highly successful entrepreneurs and business leaders. Two different speakers made powerful statements that provide insights to fuel our parenting competence.

A charismatic serial entrepreneur who has built many successful companies introduced himself with provocative self-deprecation. With a twinkle in his eye, he boasted that he had "failed his way to success." Later in the day, a warm and wise advisor to some of the wealthiest families on the planet shared his experience in helping the super-wealthy prepare their children for the responsibility of their inherited legacies. He urged the audience to "let them fail!" His advice was as jarring for a caring parent as the airline direction to put your own oxygen mask on first—but every bit as true.

Here's why.

When we approach a new challenge, we subconsciously seek advice from the three centers of our brain. We go through this internal consultation at lightning speed, but I'll slow it down for the purpose of explanation.

First, we consult our primitive brain. With grim dedication, it identifies every possible danger inherent to the task and comes back with a long list of reasons why we *should not* do it. Then we ask our emotional brain for advice, and it responds with suggestions as to how different approaches will make us (and others) feel about our actions. When we get to our cognitive brain, it often pauses for a moment before laying out rational descriptions and explanations for the wide range of approaches we might adopt, assimilating as many facts as possible to inform each alternative. Throughout this process, we send an army of little messengers into the libraries of our brain, searching for memories that might inform our deliberations. Finally, we integrate all of this information into a decision and an action plan.

In an instant, without your conscious awareness, the computer of your mind has tapped into both your own wisdom and the collective experience of your lineage that has been transferred to you through heredity and upbringing.

To be good parents, we need to allow our children the space to practice and perfect this extraordinarily complex task. In the beginning, of course, they're not at all equipped to do so, and we appropriately make all their decisions for them. But as they (and we) mature, we hopefully withdraw our control, offering merely direction and subsequently suggestion as their competence and experience grow.

Eventually, but not invariably, we stand back, allowing them to do it all on their own.

And they make mistakes! Yes, thank goodness, they make mistakes.

Before you protest, let me hasten to describe the next critical phase in the complex neurological process of decision-making. You see, the mental processing doesn't stop once we reach a decision. Instead, our brain continues to work hard, observing and documenting our progress, making corrective adjustments as necessary in order to ensure our safety and success. And, as a result, it learns so much more when we make mistakes than when we get it right.[114]

While each of us must find our own balance between guiding and watching, I would suggest that most of us parents take on too many of our children's challenges for them, denying them growth and retarding their success.

This is the paramount reason that we parents need to stand back, allowing our children to compute risk and reward for themselves. We need to allow them to make bad decisions.

Your child will need to make *many* mistakes to become a highly successful adult.

Each time we allow our children to fail, we equip them with a flood of data, eagerly stored by their primitive, emotional, and cognitive brains, increasing their computing power exponentially.

Just as important, we need to affirm them in every step of this complex journey, including (and I would say even say *especially*) when they fail. When we reprimand them for failure or poor decisions, we magnify the negative voice of their reptilian brains, making them either fearful or rebellious as they continue in their journey to adulthood.

I wish you wisdom and courage as you give your children space to take risks and fail their way to success.

CONCLUSION

BEGIN WITH
THE END IN MIND

Have you taken a big hit and abruptly found yourself down and out? Or perhaps you have slipped gradually downward until one day you woke up to the fact that you were in really bad shape.

I know I have!

Regardless of how you got there, a successful recovery always starts in the same way: Deep inside your brain, you have to decide where you're going.

Although he didn't describe the underlying neuroscience, legendary leadership guru Stephen Covey[115] knew this when he outlined his principles for effective living in *The 7 Habits of Highly Effective People*. His second habit is captured in the title of this article: "Begin with the End in Mind." He goes on to explain that we need to "envision in your mind what you cannot at present see with your eyes."[116]

A steady conversation takes place inside our heads. Each positive intention that originates in our cognitive brain has to fight its way past the protective instincts of our primitive reptilian brain. Only when the clarity, power, and durability of the positive intention overcomes the undermining questions of our protective brain is success possible.

We call this state belief. When you nourish belief, it becomes hope. When you nurture hope, it becomes reality. And so, systematically, you *real*-ize success from the inside out.

The neuroscience is simple, although not always easy. The more accurately we visualize our desired future state in our mind's eye, the better our chances are of getting there. So, if you're starting a recovery or beginning a new journey, take the time to picture your success in exquisite detail. Suffuse your cognitive brain with complete images. Co-opt every sense as you imagine the sight, sound, smell, feel, and taste of victory.

There is no doubt in my mind that this is the source of greatness. A quick look at the speeches and writings of the world's great achievers reveals the same fundamental truth:

When we describe and defend a non-negotiable image of success in our minds, we manifest it in our lives.

One of the great American scholars of the 19th century, Ralph Waldo Emerson, implicitly understood our cerebral wiring when he penned the famous inspirational statement[117]:

"The only person you are destined to become

is the person you decide to be."

Infuse your life with greatness. The journey to abundance starts in your own mind. As always, your destiny is within your reach.

A TINY GREETING
WITH HUGE IMPACT

I'm an executive coach who helps my clients achieve elite mental and physical performance. Most of my time is spent doing serious work, with serious clients. Yet, as anyone who recognizes my email sign-off knows, I always urge every one of them to "have fun!"

The reason is very simple.

Fun is a contagious positive force for you and everyone around you. Fun is good for you, even if you have significant physical, mental, or emotional challenges—or perhaps I should say *especially* if you have significant challenges!

Fun is more than an attitude. It's a physical process that starts deep in your brain. When you generate fun, have fun, or participate in fun, your body releases hormones that elevate your mood. The act of smiling alone, even if you aren't enjoying yourself, releases the feel-good hormone serotonin, which directly elevates your mood and indirectly counters the negative impacts of stress. Laughter adds even more benefits, such as improved cardiovascular health, longer life, and a stronger immune system.

This is a powerful virtuous cycle.

When you're having fun, you reach out more to others, physically and socially. Both aspects bring you health benefits. Affectionate physical contact stimulates the release of dopamine, endorphins, and oxytocin, which all work directly to elevate mood while reducing stress and anxiety. But you don't have to reach out physically to achieve these benefits; reaching out socially is also a powerful driver of emotional health. So-called "pro-social" behavior has direct benefits. This is more pronounced when you fully engage with others—and when you have fun, you take social interaction beyond a superficial connection into that territory of deep engagement. Abundant reward follows.

But what if you're not in the mood for fun? What if you're too stressed, too tired, too overwhelmed, too anything for fun?

When I suggest to someone that they "have fun," it implies that they have active control over their disposition—and that's the truth!

If we choose to, we have complete voluntary control over our thoughts. Mother Nature gave us that ability as a part of our natural wiring, gifting us a natural disposition toward health, happiness, and success. We can intentionally lead our brain toward positive, fun thoughts. You see, the negative thoughts we have are a product of our overprotective and fearful reptilian brain. But we have the power to use our cognitive brain to send more positive messages—messages focused on fun. The cognitive brain then co-opts the emotional brain, and you convert thoughts of fun into a true desire for fun. Together, the cognitive and emotional brains override any reservations harbored in the protective and conservative primitive brain. And the end result is that you actually have fun!

So, even if you don't feel in the mood for fun—and perhaps haven't felt in the mood for some time—you are still able to change your hard wiring in a positive way. If you do this often enough, for long enough, fun becomes a healthy default. After all, any behavior that you deliberately sustain for seven weeks becomes entrenched as a habit.

When I add that tiny little sentence—"Have fun!"—as a terminal greeting in all my emails and blogs, it's not a trivial, throwaway phrase. Instead, it's a heartfelt plea for each of my readers and clients to manifest a cognitive and emotional state that will bring light, health, and happiness into their own lives, and the many lives that they touch.

So don't wait…have fun!

A NOTE ABOUT COACHING

Those who invest time and energy into self-optimization know that it is difficult to fully appreciate our own inner workings.

This is why I believe that everyone who wants to succeed should have a coach—and not just any coach, but a professional coach with intimate knowledge of the human brain.

Most people I meet today understand more about the entrails of their cellular phone than the simple algorithms that drive our own natural intelligence. The outside-in and inside-out perspectives of a coach trained in neuroscience are therefore invaluable for the earnest truth-seeker. With an expert guide, you will learn to appreciate your opposing desires for safety and growth, and the rich complexity of the human psyche that plays out between these two bookends.

The emerging science relating to our own supercomputer—the human brain—is empowering. Application and mastery of these insights may soon be *the* differentiator between those who are successful and those who are not, between those who are happy and fulfilled and those who continue to struggle using old approaches even as they desperately desire new outcomes.

If you, like the many people I have written about in this book, would like to unlock the undiscovered treasure hidden in your magnificent brain, or if you are interested in finding out more about the neurocentric coaching method or attending a workshop that will help you get out of your own way and become unstoppable in life, business, relationships, parenting, or sport, please reach out to me directly through my website at www.roddycarter.com.

CONNECT

When people connect, magic happens.

This book is all about connections. These are the sparks that ignite the magic of life as we know it.

It's about intellectual, emotional, and spiritual connections that lead to deep insights. These insights, in turn, become the beacons that illuminate the path on our journey toward the truth. And it's the pursuit of truth that is our life's mission, our ultimate purpose.

Each insight that I have captured in this book has come from a connection: a chance meeting, an unexpected visitor, a story told by a client or friend, or a thought that has emerged from the great collective unconscious—the universal memory bank that mysteriously connects us to all who ever have been and those yet to travel these paths.

The energy that converts these experiences into insights is curiosity. Each of us is exposed to an enormous number of experiences on any one day. Without curiosity, each encounter would be just that: an encounter, from which we learn nothing.

The reward for a life of curiosity is the gift we call wisdom. And it is wisdom that opens the door to awareness. I believe this to be our final destination, the peak toward which we all strive: awareness of self, awareness of others, and awareness of the truths that underpin all that is, the truths that connect us all. This is consciousness, the most complete we could ever hope to be.

And it all starts with connections—so, please, reach out!

At the beginning of this book, I invited you to join me at the fireside. I invited you to rest alongside me for a moment as we paused on our great journeys. I committed to sharing some of the many insights I have enjoyed as fellow travelers have shared their wisdom with me.

Now, it's your turn. Please reach out. Share your own wisdom and curiosity with the world. Tell me your stories, or invite me to your fireplace.

You will find me at my website, www.roddycarter.com, or you can reach out to me directly by email at connect@roddycarter.com.

Yes, when people connect with curiosity, magic happens.

ADDITIONAL READING RECOMMENDATIONS

I have a special place on my bookshelf for my favorite books. This is a short selection of those that are relevant to the contents of *Fireside Wisdom* for readers looking for more inspiration and wisdom.

The Archetypes and the Collective Unconscious, Carl Jung

The Body Keeps the Score: Brain, Mind, and Body in the Healing of Trauma, Bessel van der Kolk, MD

The Book of Joy: Lasting Happiness in a Changing World, the Dalai Lama and Desmond Tutu

The Brain That Changes Itself: Stories of Personal Triumph from the Frontiers of Brain Science, Norman Doidge, MD

Homo Deus: A Brief History of Tomorrow, Yuval Noah Harari

Learned Optimism: How to Change Your Mind and Your Life, Martin E. P. Seligman

Man's Search for Meaning, Viktor E. Frankl

Mindset: The New Psychology of Success, Carol S. Dweck

Mindsight: The New Science of Personal Transformation, Daniel J. Siegel, MD

Sapiens: A Brief History of Humankind, Yuval Noah Harari

Tribe: On Homecoming and Belonging, Sebastian Junger

The Untethered Soul: The Journey beyond Yourself, Michael A. Singer

Whale Done!: The Power of Positive Relationships, Ken Blanchard

Your Brain on Nature, Eva M. Selhub and Alan C. Logan

GLOSSARY

Autosuggestion: A process in which repeated verbal messages result in a predictable outcome; e.g., if you tell yourself you are tired, you will feel tired.

Belief: Deep faith in a current or future state that compels appropriate action and makes success inevitable.

Blue space: Outdoor spaces with lots of blue, such as oceans and ponds.

Cognitive brain: The centers of the brain responsible for cognition (thought and reason); loosely centered in the cerebral cortex.

Compassion: The conversion of empathetic feelings into action.

Desire: A longing or craving for something that brings satisfaction or enjoyment.

Distress: A state of complete or partial dysfunction as a result of extreme or prolonged stress.

Elastic: The property that allows something to stretch and snap back to its original shape once the stretch-stimulus is ended.

Emotional brain: The centers of the brain (loosely equivalent to the limbic system) that are responsible for mood and instinctive behavior such as nurturing and procreation.

Empathy: Deeply experiencing the joy and pain of others.

Entitlement: An undeserved sense of self-worthiness, often found in the absence of hard work.

Eudemonic well-being: Feelings of deep emotional well-being (versus *hedonic well-being*).

Expectation: The anticipated consequences, positive or negative, for any action.

Fear: An unpleasant emotion caused by the belief that someone or something is dangerous, likely to cause pain, or a threat.

Green space: Also known as "Vitamin G"; outdoor spaces with lots of greenery, such as parks and forests.

Hedonic well-being: Superficial feelings of satisfaction (versus *eudemonic well-being*).

Learning: Adapting behavior in response to experiences.

Mood congruence: Mood's relationship with both perception and memory.

Mood diffusion: Mood spreading from one individual to another.

Neuroplasticity: The property of the brain that allows it to adapt its inner structure and function, making it pliable enough to be bent and shaped throughout our lives.

Parasympathetic nervous system: A system of nerves that carry messages to invoke relaxation.

Perceptual integration: When the Reticular Activating System (RAS) filters through sensory inputs and sends to your brain those inputs it determines to be most important.

Personal Mastery™: When we have all our organs, systems, and faculties working *for* us and are commanding our brains to serve our own interests and needs.

Phytoncides: Invisible chemicals and aromas in outdoor spaces that have health benefits.

Plastic: The property that makes something pliable, able to be bent and shaped.

Primitive (reptilian) brain: The primitive centers of the brain that are common to all reptiles and mammals and are responsible for our most primitive coping functions, such as danger avoidance, territoriality, and other rituals and behaviors that ensure survival.

Punishment: The negative consequences of an action, designed to deter the action.

Reverse empathy: The selective reinforcing of intense bonds between social allies, leading to hatred, mistrust, and hostility of anybody else.

Reward: The positive consequences of an action, designed to reinforce the action.

Self-destructive ideation: When we impose boundaries, seed doubts and fears, and sabotage our own plans.

Situational yield: Yielding to stresses and forces greater than you when it protects you and preserves your strength for more important matters.

Stress: A feeling of emotional or physical tension.

Sympathetic nervous system: A system of nerves that carry messages to invoke excitation.

Vagus nerve: A major nerve that originates in the brain and serves as the highway of the parasympathetic nervous system, inducing the "rest and digest" states.

Vulnerability: Openness, either physical or emotional, without defensiveness.

NOTES

1   Wu, T. (2014, February 6). As technology gets better, will society get worse? *The New Yorker*. https://www.newyorker.com/tech/annals-of-technology/as-technology-gets-better-will-society-get-worse

2   Shaw, C. A., & McEachern, J.C. (2001). *Toward a theory of neuroplasticity.* Taylor & Francis.

3   Doidge, N. (2007). *The brain that changes itself: Stories of personal triumph from the frontiers of brain science.* Viking.

4   Carter, R. (2015). *BodyWHealth: Journey to abundance.* Aquila Life Science Press.

5   Coue, E. (1922). *Self mastery through conscious autosuggestion: For attaining health, success and happiness.*

6   Maese, R. (2016, July 28). For Olympians, seeing (in their minds) is believing (it can happen). *The Washington Post.* https://www.washingtonpost.com/sports/olympics/for-olympians-seeing-in-their-minds-is-believing-it-can-happen/2016/07/28/6966709c-532e-11e6-bbf5-957ad17b4385_story.html

7   Goman, C. K. (2013, February 26). This is your brain on body language. *Forbes.*

8   Strack, F., Martin, L. L., & Stepper, S. (1988). Inhibiting and facilitating conditions of the human smile: A nonobtrusive test of the facial feedback hypothesis. *Journal of Personality and Social Psychology, 54*(5), 768-777.

9   Sherman, G. D., Lerner, J. S., Josephs, R. A., Renshon, J., & Gross, J. J. (2016). The interaction of testosterone and cortisol is associated with attained status in male executives. *Journal of Personality and Social Psychology, 110*(6), 921-929. https://doi.org/10.1037/pspp0000063

10   Carney, D. R., Cuddy, A. J. C., & Yap, A. J. (2010). Power posing: Brief nonverbal displays affect neuroendocrine levels and risk tolerance. *Psychological Science, 21*(10), 1363-1368.

11   Cuddy, A. (2012, June). *Your body language may shape who you are* [Video]. TED. https://www.ted.com/talks/amy_cuddy_your_body_language_may_shape_who_you_are?language=en

12   http://loni.usc.edu/about_loni/education/brain_trivia.php

13 Walter, B. L., & Shaikh, A. G. (2014). Midbrain. In M. J. Aminoff & R. B. Daroff (Eds.), *Encyclopedia of the neurological sciences, second edition* (pp. 28-33). Academic Press.

14 Garcia-Rill, E., Kezunovic, N., Hyde, J., Simon, C., Beck, P., & Urbano, F. J. (2013). Coherence and frequency in the reticular activating system (RAS). *Sleep Medicine Reviews, 17*(3), 227-238.

15 Young, G. B., & Pigott, S. E. (1999). Neurobiological basis of consciousness. *Archives of Neurology, 56*(2), 153-157. 10.1001/archneur.56.2.153.

16 Newman, J. (1995). Thalamic contributions to attention and consciousness. *Consciousness and Cognition, 4*(2), 172-193. 10.1006/ccog.1995.1024.

17 Young, G. B., & Pigott, S. E. (1999). Neurobiological basis of consciousness. *Archives of Neurology, 56*(2), 153-157. 10.1001/archneur.56.2.153.

18 Quote Investigator. (2013, January 10). *Watch your thoughts, they become words; watch your words, they become actions.* https://quoteinvestigator.com/2013/01/10/watch-your-thoughts/

19 Schaller, G. B. (1972). *The Serengeti lion: A study of predator-prey relations.* University of Chicago Press.

20 Magon, N., & Kalra, S. (2011). The orgasmic history of oxytocin: Love, lust, and labor. *Indian Journal of Endocrinology and Metabolism, 15*(Suppl 3), S156-S161.

21 Inoue, T., Yamakage, H., Tanaka, M., Kusakabe, T., Shimatsu, A., & Satoh-Asahara, N. (2019). Oxytocin suppresses inflammatory responses induced by lipopolysaccharide through inhibition of the eIF-2α–ATF4 pathway in mouse microglia. *Cells, 8*(6), 527.

22 Editors of Encyclopaedia Britannica. (2020, March 13). Vagus nerve. *Encyclopedia Britannica.* https://www.britannica.com/science/vagus-nerve

23 Pavlov, V. A., & Tracey, K. J. (2012). The vagus nerve and the inflammatory reflex—linking immunity and metabolism. *Nature Reviews Endocrinology, 8*(12), 743-754.

24 Gerritsen, R. J. S., & Band, G. H. P. (2018). Breath of life: The respiratory vagal stimulation model of contemplative activity. *Frontiers in Human Neuroscience, 12*, 397.

25   Sullivan, M. B., Erb, M., Schmalzl, L., Moonaz, S., Taylor, J. N., & Porges, S. W. (2018). Yoga therapy and polyvagal theory: The convergence of traditional wisdom and contemporary neuroscience for self-regulation and resilience. *Frontiers in Human Neuroscience.* https://doi.org/10.3389/fnhum.2018.00067

26   Hoffman, Y., & Davis, H. (2020, March 17). Sing in the shower to make friends with your vagus nerve: 7 ways to strengthen the vagus nerve and build resilience to emotional stress. *Psychology Today.* https://www.psychologytoday.com/us/blog/try-see-it-my-way/202003/sing-in-the-shower-make-friends-your-vagus-nerve

27   Kamarulzaman, N., Saleh, A. A., Hashim, S. Z., Hashim, H., & Abdul-Ghani, A. A. (2011). An overview of the influence of physical office environments towards employee. *Procedia Engineering, 20,* 262-268. https://doi.org/10.1016/j.proeng.2011.11.164

28   Wolch, J. R., Byrne, J., & Newell, J. P. (2014). Urban green space, public health, and environmental justice: The challenge of making cities 'just green enough.' *Landscape and Urban Planning, 125,* 234-244. https://doi.org/10.1016/j.landurbplan.2014.01.017; Volker, S., & Kistemann, T. (2011). The impact of blue space on human health and well-being — salutogenetic health effects of inland surface waters: A review. *International Journal of Hygiene and Environmental Health, 214*(6), 449-460. https://doi.org/10.1016/j.ijheh.2011.05.001

29   Morita, E., Fukuda, S., Nagano, J., Hamajima, N., Yamamoto, H., Iwai, Y., Nakahsima, T., Ohira, H., & Shirakawa, T. (2007). Psychological effects of forest environments on healthy adults: Shinrin-yoku (forest-air bathing, walking) as a possible method of stress reduction. *Public Health, 121*(1), 54-63. https://doi.org/10.1016/j.puhe.2006.05.024

30   Selhub, E. M., & Logan, A. C. (2014). *Your brain on nature: The science of nature's influence on your health, happiness, and vitality.* Collins.

31   Cutsuridis, V. (2013). Cognitive models of the perception-action cycle: A view from the brain. *The 2013 International Joint Conference on Neural Networks (IJCNN),* pp. 1-8. 10.1109/IJCNN.2013.6706713.

32   Thorndike, E. L. (1898). Animal intelligence: An experimental study of the associative processes in animals. *Psychological Monographs: General and Applied, 2*(4), i-109; Thorndike, E. L. (1905). *The elements of psychology.* A. G. Seiler.

33   Pavlov, I. P. (1994). *Psychopathology and psychiatry.* Routledge.

34   Stephenson-Jones, M., Floros, O., Robertson, B., & Grillner, S. (2011). Evolutionary conservation of the habenular nuclei and their circuitry controlling the dopamine and 5-hydroxytryptophan (5-HT) systems. *Proceedings of the National Academy of Sciences of the United States of America, 109*(3), 164-173. https://www.pnas.org/content/pnas/109/3/E164.full.pdf

35   Hikosaka, O., Sesack, S. R., Lecourtier, L., & Shepard, P. D. (2008). Habenula: Crossroad between the basal ganglia and the limbic system. *Journal of Neuroscience, 28*(46), 11825-11829. https://doi.org/10.1523/JNEUROSCI.3463-08.2008

36   Maia, T. V. (2009). Reinforcement learning, conditioning, and the brain: Successes and challenges. *Cognitive, Affective, & Behavioral Neuroscience, 9,* 343-364. https://link.springer.com/article/10.3758/CABN.9.4.343

37   Bromberg-Martin, E. S., & Hikosaka, O. (2011). Lateral habenula neurons signal errors in the prediction of reward information. *Nature Neuroscience, 14,* 1209-1216. https://www.nature.com/articles/nn.2902

38   Ullsperger, M., & von Cramon, D. Y. (2003). Error monitoring using external feedback: Specific roles of the habenular complex, the reward system, and the cingulate motor area revealed by functional magnetic resonance imaging. *The Journal of Neuroscience, 23*(10), 4308-4314. https://doi.org/10.1523/JNEUROSCI.23-10-04308.2003

39   Hikosaka, O. (2010). The habenula: From stress evasion to value-based decision-making. *Nature Reviews Neuroscience, 11*(7), 503-513. https://doi.org/10.1038/nrn2866

40   Wise, R. A. (2004). Dopamine, learning and motivation. *Nature Reviews Neuroscience, 5,* 483-494. https://doi.org/10.1038/nrn1406

41   Eunice Kennedy Shriver National Institute of Child Health and Human Development. (2019). What happens during sleep? *National Institutes of Health.* https://www.nichd.nih.gov/health/topics/sleep/conditioninfo/what-happens

42   Jung, C. G. (1969). *The archetypes and the collective unconscious* (2nd ed) (R. F. C. Hull, Trans.). Princeton University Press. (Original work published 1959)

43   Van der Kolk, B. A. (2014). *The body keeps the score: Brain, mind, and body in the healing of trauma*. Penguin Books.

44   Scheve, T. (2021). How many muscles does it take to smile? *Howstuffworks*. https://science.howstuffworks.com/life/inside-the-mind/emotions/muscles-smile.htm

45   Freeman, B. (2005, March 23). University of Maryland School of Medicine study shows laughter helps blood vessels function better. *World Health Net*. https://www.a4m.net/news/university_of_maryland_school_of_medicin/

46   Stevenson, S. (2012, June 25). There's magic in your smile. *Psychology Today*. https://www.psychologytoday.com/us/blog/cutting-edge-leadership/201206/there-s-magic-in-your-smile

47   Kasprak, A. (2016, December 1). Did Thomas Edison's mother lie about a letter expelling him from school? *Snopes*. https://www.snopes.com/fact-check/thomas-edisons-mom-lied-about-a-letter-expelling-her-son-from-school/

48   Conot, R. E. (2021, October 14). Thomas Edison: American Inventor. *Encyclopedia Britannica*. https://www.britannica.com/biography/Thomas-Edison

49   PetMD Editorial. (2008, September 22). Labrador retriever. *PetMD*. https://www.petmd.com/dog/breeds/c_dg_labrador_retriever

50   Peter, L. J., & Hull, R. (1969). *The Peter principle: Why things always go wrong*. William Morrow and Company.

51   Wagner, R. (2018, April 10). New evidence the Peter principle is real – and what to do about it. *Forbes*. https://www.forbes.com/sites/roddwagner/2018/04/10/new-evidence-the-peter-principle-is-real-and-what-to-do-about-it/?sh=2967ef901809

52   Editors of Encyclopaedia Britannica. (2019, May 9). Reflex. *Encyclopedia Britannica*. https://www.britannica.com/science/reflex-physiology

53 *Martin E.P. Seligman.* (n.d.). Positive Psychology Center. https://ppc.sas.upenn.edu/people/martin-ep-seligman

54 Seligman, M. E. P. (1990). *Learned optimism: How to change your mind and your life.* Vintage Books.

55 Kipling, R. (1910). If–. In *Rewards and fairies.*

56 Kirby, E. D., Muroy, S. E., Sun, W. G., Covarrubias, D., Leong, M. J., Barchas, L. A., & Kaufer, D. (2013, April 16). Acute stress enhances adult rat hippocampal neurogenesis and activation of newborn neurons via secreted astrocytic FGF2. *eLife.* https://doi.org/10.7554/eLife.00362.001

57 McKenzie, S. H., & Harris, M. F. (2013). Understanding the relationship between stress, distress and healthy lifestyle behaviour: A qualitative study of patients and general practitioners. *BMC Family Practice, 14,* 166. https://doi.org/10.1186/1471-2296-14-166

58 Kreher, J. B., & Schwartz, J. B. (2012). Overtraining syndrome: A practical guide. *Sports Health, 4*(2), 128-138. https://doi.org/10.1177/1941738111434406

59 Williams, H. L., Lubin, A., & Goodnow, J. J. (1959). Impaired performance with acute sleep loss. *Psychological Monographs: General and Applied, 73*(14), 1-26. https://doi.org/10.1037/h0093749

60 Yerkes, R. M., & Dodson, J. D. (1908). The relation of strength of stimulus to rapidity of habit-formation. *Journal of Comparative Neurology and Psychology, 18*(5), 459-482. https://doi.org/10.1002/cne.920180503

61 Matthews, G., Davies, D. R., Westerman, S. J., & Stammers, R. B. (2000). *Human performance: Cognition, stress and individual differences.* Taylor & Francis Group.

62 Hedelin, R., Wiklund, U., Bjerle, P., & Henriksson-Larsén, K. (2000). Cardiac autonomic imbalance in an overtrained athlete. *Medicine and Science in Sports and Exercise, 32*(9): 1531-1533. https://doi.org/10.1097/00005768-200009000-00001

63 Hemingway, E. (1995). *A farewell to arms.* Scribner.

64 Carter, R. (2015). *BodyWHealth: Journey to abundance.* Aquila Life Science Press.

65 Niemeyer, R. T. (Director). (1994). *Mandela: The interview* [Film].

66   Carter, R. (2015). *BodyWHealth: Journey to abundance*. Aquila Life Science Press.

67   Lombardi, V. (2021). Famous quotes by Vince Lombardi. *Vince Lombardi*. http://www.vincelombardi.com/quotes.html

68   Seligman, M. (1972). Learned helplessness. *Annual Review of Medicine, 23*, 407-412. https://doi.org/10.1146/annurev.me.23.020172.002203

69   Ibid.

70   Seligman, M. E. P., & Csikszentmihalyi, M. (2000). Positive psychology: An introduction. *American Psychologist, 55*(1), 5–14. https://doi.org/10.1037/0003-066X.55.1.5

71   https://ppc.sas.upenn.edu/

72   Seligman, M. E. P. (1990). *Learned optimism: How to change your mind and your life*. Vintage Books.

73   Seligman, M. (1972). Learned helplessness. *Annual Review of Medicine, 23*, 407-412. https://doi.org/10.1146/annurev.me.23.020172.002203

74   Stallone, S. (Director). (2006). *Rocky Balboa* [Film]. Metro-Goldwyn-Mayer, United Artists, Columbia Pictures, & Revolution Studios.

75   https://usawaterpolo.org/sports/2018/12/19/junior-olympics.aspx

76   Wild, B., Erb, M., & Bartels, M. (2001). Are emotions contagious? Evoked emotions while viewing emotionally expressive faces: Quality, quantity, time course and gender differences. *Psychiatry Research, 102*(2), 109-124. https://doi.org/10.1016/S0165-1781(01)00225-6

77   Forgas, J. P, & Eich, E. (2013). Affective influences on cognition: Mood congruence, mood dependence, and mood effects on processing strategies. In A. F. Healy, R. W. Proctor, & I. B. Weiner (Eds.), *Handbook of psychology: Experimental psychology* (pp. 61–82). John Wiley & Sons, Inc.

78   Scheve, T. (2021). How many muscles does it take to smile? *Howstuffworks*. https://science.howstuffworks.com/life/inside-the-mind/emotions/muscles-smile.htm

79   Root, A. A., & Stephens, J. A. (2003). Organization of the central control of muscles of facial expression in man. *The Journal of Physiology, 549*(1), 289-298. https://doi.org/10.1113/jphysiol.2002.035691

80 Du, S., Tao, Y., & Martinez, A. M. (2015). Compound facial expressions of emotion. *Proceedings of the National Academy of Sciences of the United States of America, 111*(15), 1454-1462. https://doi.org/10.1073/pnas.1322355111

81 Wood, A., Rychlowska, M., Korb, S., & Niedenthal, P. (2016). Fashioning the face: Sensorimotor simulation contributes to facial expression recognition. *Trends in Cognitive Sciences, 20*(3), 227-240. https://doi.org/10.1016/j.tics.2015.12.010

82 Strean, W. B. (2009). Laughter prescription. *Canadian Family Physician, 55*(10), 965-967.

83 Kraft, T. L., & Pressman, S. D. (2012). Grin and bear it: The influence of manipulated facial expression on the stress response. *Psychological Science, 23*(11), 1372-1378 https://doi.org/10.1177/0956797612445312

84 Darwin, C. (1872). *The expressions of the emotions in man and animals.* John Murray.

85 Söderkvist, S., Ohlén, K., & Dimberg, U. (2018). How the experience of emotion is modulated by facial feedback. *Journal of Nonverbal Behavior, 42*(1), 129-151. https://dx.doi.org/10.1007%2Fs10919-017-0264-1

86 Reis, H. T., Wilson, I. M., Monestere, C., Bernstein, S., Clark, K., Seidl, E., Franco, M., Gioioso, E., Freeman, L., & Radoane, K. (1990). What is similing is beautiful and good. *European Journal of Social Psychology, 20*(3), 259-267. https://doi.org/10.1002/ejsp.2420200307

87 Papa, A., & Bonanno, G. A. (2008). Smiling in the face of adversity: The interpersonal and intrapersonal functions of smiling. *Emotion, 8*(1), 1-12. https://doi.org/10.1037/1528-3542.8.1.1

88 Abel, E. L., & Kruger, M. L. (2010). Smile intensity in photographs predicts longevity. *Psychological Science, 21*(4), 542-544. https://doi.org/10.1177/0956797610363775

89 Barrie, J. M. (2011). *Peter and Wendy.* Charles Scribner's Sons.

90 Addyman, C., & Addyman, I. (2014). The science of baby laughter. *Comedy Studies, 4*(2), 143-153. https://doi.org/10.1386/cost.4.2.143_1

91   Gerloff, P. (2011, June 21). You're not laughing enough, and that's no joke. *Psychology Today*. https://www.psychologytoday.com/us/blog/the-possibility-paradigm/201106/youre-not-laughing-enough-and-thats-no-joke

92   Martin, R. A., & Kuiper, N. A. (1999). Daily occurrence of laughter: Relationships with age, gender, and Type A personality. *Humor, 12*(4), 355-384. https://doi.org/10.1515/humr.1999.12.4.355

93   Scott, S., Lavan, N., Chen, S., & McGettigan, C. (2014). The social life of laughter. *Trends in Cognitive Science, 18*(12), 618-620. https://dx.doi.org/10.1016%2Fj.tics.2014.09.002

94   Mora-Ripoll, R. (2010). The therapeutic value of laughter in medicine. *Alternative Therapies in Health & Medicine, 16*(6), 56-64.

95   Bennett, M. P., & Lengacher, C. (2008). Humor and laughter may influence health: III. Laughter and health outcomes. *Evidence-based Complementary and Alternative Medicine, 5*(1), 37-40. https://doi.org/10.1093/ecam/nem041

96   Sakai, Y., & Takayanagi, K. (2013). A trial of improvement of immunity in cancer patients by laughter therapy. *Japan Hospitals: The Journal of Japan Hospital Association, 32*, 53-59.

97   Smith, M., & Segal, J. (2014). Laughter is the best medicine. *Humor and Health, 7*(2). http://www.pitwm.net/Humor_And_Health.pdf

98   Ibid.

99   Ibid.

100 https://isaworlds.com/adaptive/2017/en/

101 http://brenebrown.com/

102 Shamay-Tsoory, S. G. (2011). The neural bases for empathy. *The Neuroscientist, 17*(1), 18-24. https://doi.org/10.1177%2F1073858410379268

103 De Sousa, A., McDonald, S., Rushby, J., Li, S., Dimoska, A., & James, C. (2011). Understanding deficits in empathy after traumatic brain injury: The role of affective responsivity. *Cortex, 47*(5), 526-535. https://doi.org/10.1016/j.cortex.2010.02.004

104 Simas, E. N., Clifford, S., & Kirkland, J. H. (2020). How empathic concern fuels political polarization. *American Political Science Review, 114*(1), 258-269. https://doi.org/10.1017/S0003055419000534

105 Brown, J. (2006). *A leader's guide to reflective practice.* Trafford Publishing.

106 Kandel, E. R., Barres, B. A., & Hudspeth, A. J. (2013). Nerve cells, neural circuitry, and behavior. In E. R. Kandel, J. H. Schwartz, T. M. Jessell, S. A. Siegelbaum, & A. J. Hudspeth (Eds.), *Principles of neural science* (5th ed.) (pp. 21-38). McGraw-Hill.

107 Brooks, A. W., Dai, H., & Schweitzer, M. E. (2014). I'm sorry about the rain! Superfluous apologies demonstrate empathic concern and increase trust. *Social Psychological and Personality Science, 5*(4), 467-474.

108 Lewicki, R. J., Polin, B., & Lount Jr., R. B. (2016). An exploration of the structure of effective apologies. *Negotiation and Conflict Management Research, 9*(2), 177-196.

109 Burton, L. R. (2020). The neuroscience and positive impact of gratitude in the workplace. *The Journal of Medical Practice Management, 35*(4), 215-218.

110 Creswell, J. D., Dutcher, J. M., Klein, W. M. P., Harris, P. R., & Levine, J. M. (2013). Self-affirmation improves problem-solving under stress. *PLoS One, 8*(5). https://doi.org/10.1371/journal.pone.0062593

111 Mander, G. (1991). Some thoughts on sibling rivalry and competitiveness. *British Journal of Psychotherapy, 7*(4), 368-379. https://doi.org/10.1111/j.1752-0118.1991.tb01142.x

112 Godfray, H. C. J. (1995). Signaling of need between parents and young: Parent-offspring conflict and sibling rivalry. *The American Naturalist, 146*(1). https://doi.org/10.1086/285784

113 Leung, A. K. D., & Robson, W. L. M. (1991). Sibling rivalry. *Clinical Pediatrics, 30*(5), 314-317. https://doi.org/10.1177%2F000992289103000510

114 Chialvo, D. R., & Bak, P. (1999). Learning from mistakes. *Neuroscience, 90*(4), 1137-1148. https://doi.org/10.1016/S0306-4522(98)00472-2

115 https://www.stephencovey.com/

116 Covey, S. R. (1989). *The 7 habits of highly effective people.* Free Press.

117 Emerson, R. W. (1841). *Essays: First series.*